Immunology Nomenclature
Turner/Natvig (Editors)

Publication of this work was supported by an unrestricted educational grant from Serotec Ltd., Kidlington, Oxford, UK.

Publication of this work was supported by an unrestricted educational grant from PharMingen, San Diego, CA, USA.

Immunology Nomenclature

Edited by
Malcolm W. Turner and Jacob B. Natvig

This publication is appearing as Supplement 2 (1998) to *The Immunologist*

Hogrefe & Huber Publishers
Seattle · Toronto · Bern · Göttingen

Library of Congress Cataloging-in-Publication Data

is available via the Library of Congress Marc Database under the

LC Catalog Card Number 98-73937.

Canadian Cataloguing in Publication Data

Main entry under title:
Immunology nomenclature

ISBN 0-88937-208-X

1. Immunology – Nomenclature. I. Natvig, Jacob B. II. Turner, M.W.
QR180.4.I45 1999 571.9'6'014 C98-932162-2

USA: P.O. Box 2487, Kirkland, WA 98083-2487
Phone (425) 820-1500, Fax (425) 823-8324
CANADA: 12 Bruce Park Avenue, Toronto, Ontario M4P 2S3
Phone (416) 482-6339
SWITZERLAND: Länggass-Strasse 76, CH-3000 Bern 9
Phone (031) 300-4500, Fax (031) 300-4590
GERMANY: Rohnsweg 25, D-37085 Göttingen
Phone (0551) 49609-0, Fax (0551) 49609-88

Printed and bound in Germany
ISBN 0-88937-208-X

Table of Contents

Preface

The science of immunology underwent a major transition in the early 1960's as the structure and function of antibody molecules was unravelled and it became possible to describe in fine detail the relationships between the heterogeneous proteins with such biological activity. In 1964 the World Health Organization (WHO) convened a meeting in Prague on Nomenclature of Human Immunoglobulins and the set of recommended guidelines which was published became the first of a series in the area of immunology. The urgent need for such recommendations was underscored by the fact that in 1964 five alternative notations were in use to describe IgG, with four alternatives used for IgM. Many of the names in use at this time reflected the size and charge characteristics of the proteins.

The WHO International Reference Centre for Immunoglobulins in Lausanne subsequently coordinated documents covering genetic factors of immunoglobulins, human immunoglobulin subclasses and immunoglobulin E. Documents on the proteins of the complement system and factors of the HLA system were also generated at this time under the auspices of WHO.

In 1971 the International Union of Immunological Societies (IUIS) was founded and a Standing Committee on Nomenclature established. Since its inception this Committee has approved documents covering nomenclature in a wide range of immunological areas. In most cases these documents are prepared by a subcommittee of experts working in particular specialized areas which may meet both formally and informally at international conferences, but mostly operate by exchanging numerous drafts until a consensus view emerges. The proposals of such subcommittees are then considered by the members of the Standing Committee and, if approved, go forward for publication in the *Bulletin of the World Health Organization.* The Standing Committee has always encouraged wide dissemination of these documents and Editors of the major immunological titles receive copies for inclusion in their journals.

More than thirty nomenclature documents have been published since 1964, and the Council of IUIS was of the opinion that immunologists might find it useful to have all this material gathered together in a single reference volume. The present publication arises from that decision. The documents appear in their original format but, to facilitate searching, the material has been grouped into ten general clusters. These are: (A) Immunoglobulins (B) T cell receptor genes (C) HLA antigens (D) Fc receptors (E) Complement proteins (F) Interleukins (G) CD antigens (H) Leukocyte locomotion proteins (I) Allergens and (J) Amyloid proteins. Within any one cluster the documents are reprinted in chronological sequence in order to provide continuity. This should be helpful to readers when provisional (or workshop) designations have been superseded by another name in a later document, or when the scope of the nomenclature has been extended without reduplication of the original documents.

Scientific nomenclature is a very important issue. It helps to minimize ambiguities in the literature and improve the precision with which scientists communicate with each other. The field of immunology seems to be particularly over-supplied with acronyms and in-house jargon. However, progress can be difficult and there are frequently prolonged arguments about the fine details before agreement is reached. Occasionally a problem arises where a nomenclature already exists and is designed to permit extension in the future, e.g., the interleukins. It is absolutely imperative that additions to such series are not proposed unilaterally by individual scientists or groups but are submitted to the appropriate subcommittee for international evaluation and agreement.

At present there are sixteen sub-committees dealing with various aspects of immunological nomenclature including Allergens (chairperson: H. Løwenstein), Chemokines (R. Thorpe), CD antigens (S. F. Schlossman), Collectins (M. W. Turner), Complement (D. T. Fearon), Fc receptors (J. P. Kinet) and Interleukins (J. Schrader). The Standing Committee always welcomes suggestions for additional topics which need to be addressed and these should be sent to the Chairman (details below). The approval of agreed nomenclature is one of the major tasks of IUIS and it is hoped that this supplement will not only provide immunologists with valuable reference material but also serve to focus attention on the importance of this IUIS function.

M. W. Turner
Chairman, WHO/IUIS Nomenclature Committee
Immunobiology Unit, Institute of Child Health
University College London
30 Guilford Street, London WC1N 1EH, UK
Fax: +44 171 813 8494, e-mail: m.turner@ich.ucl.ac.uk

J. B. Natvig
Editor-in-Chief, *The Immunologist*
Institute of Immunology and Rheumatology
Fr. Qvamsgt. 1, N-0172 Oslo, Norway
Fax +47 22 200636, e-mail: j.b.natvig@rh.uio.no

Acknowledgments

The Editors are grateful to Dr Julia Bodmer for permission to reprint the Nomenclature for Factors of the HLA System 1996 and to Dr Steven Marsh for proofreading this contribution.

The other documents contained in this collection were originally published in the following sources and are reproduced here with permission of the World Health Organization:

Cluster	No.	Title
A	1	Nomenclature for human immunoglobulins. *Bull Wld Hlth Org* 1964; 30:447–450
A	2	Notation for genetic factors of human immunoglobulins. *Bull Wld Hlth Org* 1965; 33:721–724
A	3	Notation for human immunoglobulin subclasses. *Bull Wld Hlth Org* 1966; 35:953
A	4	Immunoglobulin E, a new class of human immunoglobulin. *Bull Wld Hlth Org* 1968; 38:151–152
C	5	Nomenclature for factors of the HL-A system. *Bull Wld Hlth Org* 1968; 39:483–486
E	6	Nomenclature of complement. *Bull Wld Hlth Org* 1968; 39:935–938
A	7	An extension of the nomenclature for immunoglobulins. *Bull Wld Hlth Org* 1969; 41:975–978
C	8	Nomenclature for factors of the HL-A system. *Bull Wld Hlth Org* 1972; 47:659–662
A	9	Nomenclature for human immunoglobulins. *Bull Wld Hlth Org* 1973; 48:373
C	10	Nomenclature for factors of the HLA system, 1977. *Bull Wld Hlth Org* 1978; 56:461–465
A	11	Proposed rules for the designation of immunoglobulins of animal origin. *Bull Wld Hlth Org* 1978; 56:815–817
H	12	A proposal for the definition of terms related to locomotion of leukocytes and other cells. *Bull Wld Hlth Org* 1980; 58:505–509
C	13	Nomenclature for factors of the HLA system, 1980. *Bull Wld Hlth Org* 1980; 58:945–948
E	14	Nomenclature of the alternative activating pathway of complement. *Bull Wld Hlth Org* 1981; 59:489–491
G	15	Nomenclature for clusters of differentiation (CD) of antigens defined on human leukocyte populations. *Bull Wld Hlth Org* 1984; 62:809–811
C	16	Nomenclature for factors of the HLA system, 1984. *Bull Wld Hlth Org* 1985; 63:399
I	17	Allergen nomenclature. *Bull Wld Hlth Org* 1986; 64:767–770
D	18	Nomenclature of the Fc receptors. *Bull Wld Hlth Org* 1989; 67:449
A	19	Nomenclature for synthetic peptides respresentative of immunoglobulin chain sequences. *Bull Wld Hlth Org* 1990; 68:109–111
F	20	Nomenclature for secreted regulatory proteins of the immune system (interleukins). *Bull Wld Hlth Org* 1991; 69: 483–484
E	21	Nomenclature for human complement component C2. *Bull Wld Hlth Org* 1992; 70:527–528
E	22	Revised nomenclature for human complement component C4. *Bull Wld Hlth Org* 1992; 70:531–535
E	23	Nomenclature for human complement factor B. *Bull Wld Hlth Org* 1992; 70:541–543
J	24	Nomenclature of amyloid and amyloidosis. *Bull Wld Hlth Org* 1993; 71:105–108
B	25	Nomenclature for T-cell receptor (TCR) gene segments of the immune system. *Bull Wld Hlth Org* 1993; 71:113–115
I	26	Allergen nomenclature. *Bull Wld Hlth Org* 1994; 72:797–806
D	27	Nomenclature of Fc receptors. *Bull Wld Hlth Org* 1994; 72:809
G	28	CD antigens 1993: An updated nomenclature for clusters of differentiation on human cells. *Bull Wld Hlth Org* 1994; 72:807–808

F	29	Nomenclature for secreted regulatory proteins of the immune system (interleukins): Update. *Bull Wld Hlth Org* 1994; 72:811
F	30	Interleukin-16. *Bull Wld Hlth Org* 1996; 74:451
F	31	Nomenclature for secreted regulatory proteins of the immune system (Interleukins): Update. *Bull Wld Hlth Org* 1997 75:175
G	32	CD antigens 1996: Updated nomenclature for clusters of differentiation on human cells. *Bull Wld Hlth Org* 1997; 75: 385–387
C	33	Nomenclature for Factors of the HLA System, 1996 (published independently of IUIS)
A	34	Nomenclature of immunoglobulin A and other proteins of the mucosal immune system. *Bull Wld Hlth Org* 1998; 76: 427–428

Nomenclature for Human Immunoglobulins *

Definition of immunoglobulins

Immunoglobulins are proteins of animal origin endowed with known antibody activity, and certain proteins related to them by chemical structure and hence antigenic specificity. Related proteins for which antibody activity has not been demonstrated are included—for example, myeloma proteins, Bence-Jones proteins and naturally occurring subunits of the immunoglobulins.

Immunoglobulins are not restricted to the plasma but may be found in other body fluids or tissues, such as urine, spinal fluid, lymph-nodes, spleen, etc. Proteins may occur which fulfil the above requirements but which have widely differing physicochemical properties such as electrophoretic mobility, sedimentation coefficient, and diffusion coefficient, and different chemical properties such as carbohydrate content, amino-acid composition of polypeptide chains, etc. Immunoglobulins do not include the components of the complement system.

Terminology

Advances in biological and chemical studies of immunoglobulins have emphasized the need for a nomenclature and classification to meet new requirements. Terminology should be based on the identification of the polypeptide chains which by complementation make up the molecule. This principle should allow a precise description of different molecules. In addition, broader terms are needed for grouping classes of molecules with common physicochemical and biological characteristics. This can be achieved by minor modifications of current terminologies.

The following notation for immunoglobulins provides:

(*a*) an abbreviated notation to designate the major classes of immunoglobulins;

(*b*) terms to designate the polypeptide chains of the immunoglobulin molecules.

Whenever possible terms already in common usage have been retained.

Abbreviated notation

Two symbols for immunoglobulins are considered to be appropriate. The logical abbreviation for the term immunoglobulin would be the symbol Ig. Since the symbol Ig may present some difficulties in verbal communication and, furthermore, since the symbol γ has been commonly employed to designate the immunoglobulins, both symbols γ and Ig are recognized as appropriate. These symbols should be accompanied by a capital letter designating a specific class of immunoglobulin, for example, γG, γM . . . IgG, IgM . . ., as noted below. The symbol should *not* be followed by arabic numbers, which in the past have been used to indicate electrophoretic mobilities.

The following symbols proposed for major classes of immunoglobulin molecules are based on differences associated with heavy chains.

Present usage	*Proposed usage*
γ, 7Sγ, 6.6Sγ, γ_2, γ_{ss}	γG or IgG
β_2A, γ_1A	γA or IgA
γ_1M, β_2M, 19Sγ, γ-macroglobulin	γM or IgM

The following symbols are proposed for types of molecules identified by the properties of light chains.

Present usage	*Proposed usage*
Type I, 1, B	Type K
Type II, 2, A	Type L

Notation for polypeptide chains

Two major groups of polypeptide chains are now recognized as occurring in immunoglobulin molecules:

(*a*) The L or B chains (Mol. wt. about 20 000) are at this time the only subunits known to be common to the three major classes of immunoglobulins;

(*b*) The H or A chains (Mol. wt. about 50 000) determine the distinctive properties of each class.

It is suggested that the terms L and H, and A and B to denote chains be discarded, in view of the more precise terminology proposed below. For simplicity, however, it is advisable to designate two major groups of polypeptide chains by the terms " light " and " heavy ". The designation of these polypeptide chains may be revised as new evidence accumulates. For example, the possibility that the

* This memorandum was drafted by the signatories (see pages 449-450) following discussions held during the WHO Meeting on Nomenclature of Human Immunoglobulins that took place on 29-30 May 1964 in Prague, just before the International Symposium on the Cellular and Molecular Basis of Antibody Formation.

Requests for reprints should be addressed to: Immunology, World Health Organization, Palais des Nations, Geneva, Switzerland.

" heavy " chain is in fact several chains has been considered. Until definite proof of this hypothesis that the heavy chain is composed of two or more chains is provided, the heavy chain will be considered as a single chain in the following description.

(*a*) *Heavy chains.* It is proposed that the heavy chains be designated by small Greek letters corresponding to the Roman capital letters used for the immunoglobulin classes.

Immunoglobulin class	*Heavy chain*
γG or IgG	γ (gamma)
γA or IgA	α (alpha)
γM or IgM	μ (mu)

It is recognized that the symbol γ has been used in two different designations. No ambiguity should occur, however, since γ is not used alone in either case. The symbol is always used in association with either the word immunoglobulin or chain, for example:

" γG-immunoglobulin " for the class of immunoglobulin, and

" γ-chain " for the polypeptide chain.

Use of the term γ-chain (rather than another Greek letter) to designate the heavy chain of the IgG or γG-immunoglobulin molecule preserves an association with the distinctive properties of this major component within the immunoglobulin system.

(*b*) *Light chains.* Two forms of light chain (Type I and Type II) are recognized as occurring in man. To conform with the use of Greek letters for distinctive polypeptide chains, the following symbols are proposed:

Present usage	*Proposed usage* — *Abbreviated notation for immunoglobulins*	*Proposed usage* — *Notation for light chains*
Type I	Type K	κ (kappa)
Type II	Type L	λ (lambda)

(*c*) *Molecular formulae.* The proposed system is similar to that in use for haemoglobin. Some typical formulae would be:

Present usage	*Abbreviated notation for immunoglobulins*	*Molecular formulae*
7Sγ - type I	γGK or IgGK	$\gamma_2\ \kappa_2$
7Sγ - type II	γGL or IgGL	$\gamma_2\ \lambda_2$
γ_1A - type I	γAK or IgAK	$\alpha_2\ \kappa_2$
γ_1A - type II	γAL or IgAL	$\alpha_2\ \lambda_2$
γ_1M - type I	γMK or IgMK	$(\mu_2\ \kappa_2)n$ *
γ_1M - type II	γML or IgML	$(\mu_2\ \lambda_2)n$ *
Urinary globulin composed of light chains		κ_2 and λ_2 (if in the dimer form)

* n in this case may be 6.

If it is desirable to indicate that the protein is a myeloma protein, Bence-Jones protein, etc., this information can be added in parentheses after the formula.

Classes and subclasses

There may be different degrees of molecular association within an immunoglobulin class, and this distinction may be made by the terms dimers, trimers and polymers of a particular unit. In addition the sedimentation coefficient or the molecular weight may be cited.

It may become necessary to recognize a new class of immunoglobulins when molecules containing a novel heavy chain are discovered. This new heavy chain should differ from the presently known heavy chains to the same extent that the latter differ from one another. Similar principles should be applied to the differentiation of new light chains. When new polypeptide chains are characterized, they should be designated with a new small letter of the Greek alphabet. If new immunoglobulins contain chains which can be recognized as members of presently known classes even though they differ in some significant detail, then it may become necessary to define them as new *subclasses.* Until adequate characterization of such novel polypeptide chains is achieved, it is suggested that a non-committal designation be used, and enclosed in parentheses as illustrated below. Terms indicative of origin, such as geographical names and the names of patients, could be used. For example, a newly found immunoglobulin with the characteristics of class G, thought to be a new subclass, if identified in Prague, could be designated IgG(Pr). If several such components are identified simultaneously, a combination of abbreviated words and numbers could be used—γG(Pr-1), γG(Pr-2), etc.

When new immunoglobulins, which can be recognized as subclasses, have been well characterized, they will be indicated by the symbol of the major class followed by a small Roman letter (IgAa, IgAb), to be read as A subclass a. Similarly, the new chain responsible for the subclass should be indicated as αa, αb, etc.

The WHO Reference Centre for Immunoglobulins is being established at the Institute of Biochemistry, Lausanne, Switzerland, and investigators are encouraged to consult the Centre concerning notation of new immunoglobulins.

Fragments

The term " fragment " is reserved for portions of the molecule obtained as a result of the cleavage of peptide bonds. Proteolytic enzymes produce heterogeneous groups of fragments which nevertheless can be distinguished by immunological and chemical properties. It is useful to name these fragments, but it is stressed that a single designation does not imply homogeneity.

Fragments produced by digestion with papain

Present usage	*Proposed usage*
A, C, S (I, II) *	Fab-fragment (antigen-binding)
B, F (III) *	Fc-fragment (crystallizable)
A piece	Fd-fragment

* The parentheses enclose terms used for fragments in the rabbit.

If it is necessary to specify the chain from which fragments are derived, the name of the chain may be subscripted—for example, Fcγ or Fdγ. For 5S fragments obtained by pepsin digestion and having two antibody sites, the notation would be $F(ab')_2$. The univalent pepsin fragments should be designated as Fab′. If possible details of molecular formulae may be appended. For fragments derived from immunoglobulins without known antibody activity, the same notation should be used.

Immunoglobulins in proliferative disorders of lymphocytic or plasmacytic cells

It is suggested that the distinctive proteins related to the immunoglobulins be classified as " discrete components " or " pathological proteins ", and that they be classified further in relation to the corresponding normal protein. It is recognized that at this time no decision can be made as to whether these are large amounts of normally present immunoglobulins or abnormal proteins related to them.

In the abbreviated notation, these proteins should not be classified precisely in the absence of an appropriate clinical diagnosis. In patients with multiple myeloma or macroglobulinaemia they should be termed: (*a*) G myeloma or A myeloma globulin; (*b*) M-macroglobulin (Waldenström); (*c*) light-chain protein or Bence-Jones protein depending on the thermosolubility properties associated with them; (*d*) heavy-chain proteins with the appropriate class designation.

As is the case for normal immunoglobulins, the notation for polypeptide chains can be used regardless of the disease process with which they are associated. This provides for those instances where relatively homogeneous immunoglobulins are associated with pathological states other than those mentioned above. Under those circumstances the diagnosis can be listed separately.

Nomenclature of immunoglobulins in other species

In the nomenclature of immunoglobulins of different species, it is recommended that the same principles used in devising a nomenclature for human immunoglobulins be applied. As many criteria as possible, for example, immunological cross-reactivity, estimation of molecular weight, carbohydrate content and biological properties, should be employed to establish whatever similarities in chemical structure may exist between animal and human immunoglobulin classes.

For example, in animal sera the use of γM or IgM is recommended for a class of immunoglobulins with molecular weight of the order of magnitude of 10^6. In addition, other properties of the human γM or IgM—such as high carbohydrate content, dissociation by mercaptoethanol, and antigenic relationship—should be considered.

Notation for genes, genotypes and allotypes

As a logical consequence of the criteria followed for outlining the above proposed terminology, the gene notation should be based on the specification of the molecular subunit controlled by the gene in question. For immunoglobulins, unusual genetic situations may occur, such as somatic mutation, repeats, etc., posing problems which at the moment cannot be precisely foreseen. Moreover, identification of individual variants under genetic control has been limited until now to variants detected by serological reagents (Gm groups, allotypes). The problem of genetic terms related to immunoglobulins, as well as terms for serological variants, would best be dealt with by a committee of investigators active in the field of immunoglobulins, and representing different disciplines (genetics, immunology, protein chemistry).

* * *

R. Ceppellini, Institute of Medical Genetics, University of Turin, Turin, Italy
S. Dray, Laboratory of Immunology, National Institutes of Health, Bethesda, Md., USA
G. Edelman, The Rockefeller Institute, New York, N.Y., USA

J. Fahey, National Cancer Institute, National Institutes of Health, Bethesda, Md., USA
F. Franěk, Department of Immunology, Institute of Microbiology of the ČSSR Academy of Sciences, Prague, Czechoslovakia
E. Franklin, New York University College of Medicine, New York, N.Y., USA
H. C. Goodman, Immunology, World Health Organization, Geneva, Switzerland
P. Grabar, Institut Pasteur, Paris, France
A. E. Gurvich, Institute of Biological and Medical Chemistry, USSR Academy of Medical Sciences, Moscow, USSR
J. F. Heremans, Cliniques universitaires St Pierre, University of Louvain, Louvain, Belgium
H. Isliker, University of Lausanne, Institute of Biochemistry, Lausanne, Switzerland
F. Karush, Department of Microbiology, University of Pennsylvania School of Medicine, Philadelphia, Pa., USA
E. Press, Department of Immunology, Wright-Fleming Institute of Microbiology, London, England
Z. Trnka, Immunology, World Health Organization, Geneva, Switzerland

NOTATION FOR GENETIC FACTORS OF HUMAN IMMUNOGLOBULINS *

In a previous memorandum stating recommendations for a uniform notation for human immunoglobulins [a] it was considered advisable that analogous recommendations be made in the future for genes, genotypes and allotypes. In that memorandum, classes of human immunoglobulins which are common to all normal individuals of a given species were considered. These classes of immunoglobulins can be distinguished from each other by a number of means including their antigenic specificity (isotypic specificity).

Another kind of classification, which is at present based on serological typing, distinguishes variants which occur among proteins of the above classes. The corresponding determinants, which are present in some groups of individuals within the species, define antigenic specificities which in animals are commonly termed as " allotypic specificities " and in man as " factors ". Many of these antigenic specificities determine genetic polymorphisms in the different races of man and other animals.

The genetic factors of human immunoglobulins are currently identified by serological tests which measure the inhibition by the test material of the agglutination of erythrocytes pre-coated with incomplete antibody. The agglutinating antibodies occur in selected sera from patients with rheumatoid arthritis or from normal subjects. The incomplete coating antibodies are usually IgG immunoglobulin molecules and the agglutinating reagents are usually IgM molecules. The whole serum, an isolated immunoglobulin, or an immunoglobulin subunit may be used in such an inhibition test.

The term " factor " defines a particular property of certain immunoglobulins which enables them to be identified by a given set of reagents, but it should be noted that the characterization of factors by these means does not preclude the possibility of a cross-reaction.

* This memorandum was drafted by the signatories (see last page) following discussions held during the meeting of the WHO Scientific Group on Genes, Genotypes and Allotypes of Immunoglobulins, that took place from 31 May to 5 June 1965 in Geneva. A French version will be published in a later issue.

[a] *Bull. Wld Hlth Org.*, 1964, **30**, 447-450.

Family studies have shown that the factors involved are inherited according to Mendelian principles. Two series of factors controlled by independent genetic systems are known; one (the Gm system) is associated with the heavy polypeptide chain of some IgG molecules, and the other (the Inv system) is associated with light polypeptide chains of immunoglobulin molecules.

The nomenclature currently in use is based on serological tests, with genetical analysis providing linkage group information. In higher organisms, the term locus (and the corresponding terminology for genes and genotypes) may be ambiguously used for indicating either a complex chromosomal region or a structural gene, and owing to the nature of serological analysis a one-to-one correspondence between one factor and one gene or one region of a gene cannot be inferred at the present time. For these reasons, the term " system " is used here for a unit of closely linked genetic information which cannot be separated into subunits at the level of resolution allowed by formal human genetics.

A new notation should provide a symbol which suggests the relation of the system to the structure it influences, which does not go beyond established fact and which is sufficiently flexible to meet future needs. It should relate to prior terminology for the same system if at all possible, and provide for different systems a series of symbols which differ from each other by at least two letters when practicable. The following recommendations have been designed to meet these requirements as far as possible.

Notation for the factors of the Gm and Inv systems

At the present time, the accumulated information is insufficient to permit precise correlation of the genetic loci for the human immunoglobulins with the structures they influence. Consequently, it seems advisable at this time to retain the present symbols Gm and Inv to describe the two currently recognized systems. For these systems, particularly at the Gm locus, an ever-increasing complexity has been developing in recent years. To avoid these complexities and the implication of possibly false relationships, we recommend a non-committal, flexible numerical notation, similar to that suggested for the *Salmonella* antigens, Rh blood groups, and histocompatibility antigens in the mouse.

The assignment of numbers to the already known Gm and Inv factors has been done using the principles outlined below and considering also the order of their discovery and the known relationships of the Gm factors to the subgroups of the polypeptide chain of IgG.

Notation for the factors at the Gm locus *

Original	*New*
a	1
x	2
b^w and b^2	3
f	4
b and b^1	5
c	6
r	7
e	8
p	9
b^α	10
b^β	11
b^γ	12
b^3	13
b^4	14

Notation for the factors at the Inv locus

Original	*New*
1 (lower-case L)	1
a	2
b	3

* A number has not been assigned to Gm (D) because it has been found to be an artefact and not a Gm factor.

Either of two methods is suitable for recording the phenotype of an individual:

(*a*) Record the result obtained with each set of reagents: e.g., Gm(1,−2,3,4,5); Inv (1,−2,3). Punctuation includes commas between the reactions with each set of reagents. This would mean that the sample was tested with reagents which correspond to the factors Gm(1), Gm(2), Gm(3), Gm(4), and Gm(5) and Inv(1), Inv(2), and Inv(3); and that it was positive with the test systems for Gm(1), Gm(3), Gm(4), and Gm(5), and negative for Gm(2); and positive for Inv(1) and (3), and negative for Inv(2).

(*b*) Record only the positive results: e.g., Gm(1,3, 4,5); Inv(1,3). In this case, the factors tested cannot be determined from the recorded phenotype and reference must be made to the list of reagents used for this information.

It is recognized that studies with several sets of reagents of Gm factors 7-14 inclusive have not yet been extensively published. Nor is the closeness of the relationship between Gm3 and Gm4 precisely known at the present time. These factors have nevertheless been assigned separate numbers here. Future decisions in the form of deletions of some numbers are foreseen.

The phenotypes of isolated discrete (e.g.,myeloma) proteins may be recorded on the same basis as whole serum and by adding the symbol for the immunoglobulin subtype if known. For example: phenotypes

γ_2b:Gm(1,2); or γWe:Gm(1,2); κ:Inv(1); etc.

Notation for genes

Symbols for genes should be underlined when typed and italicized when printed. The factors determined by the gene should be indicated by superscript digits.

It is understood that the assignment of a genotype to a phenotype can be done only after genetic analysis, i.e., the observation of family segregation. Assignment of " the most probable " genotype in the absence of family data should be clearly indicated.

Examples

Phenotype *	*Population*	*Most probable genotype*
Gm(1,5)	Caucasoid	Gm^1/Gm^5
Gm(1,5)	Negroid	$Gm^{1,5}/Gm^{1,5}$
Gm(1,2)	Caucasoid or Mongoloid	$Gm^{1,2}/Gm^{1,2}$ or $Gm^{1,2}/Gm^1$

* All samples were tested for Gm(1), Gm(2) and Gm(5).

It should be emphasized that findings in other immunological systems indicate that serological specificities may appear in the phenotype which may not be represented in the genotype (that is, specificities resulting from interaction of different genes). Although such specificities have not yet been found in the human immunoglobulins, the proposed system of nomenclature may be used to record them.

The use of genetic symbols containing several numbers is a convenient notation to describe the inheritance of complex patterns of serological reactions (phenogroups). The symbols do not imply that regions corresponding to the *individual* numbers do or do not exist in the relevant genes. For example, a gene $Gm^{1,2}$ does not necessarily have part of its structure determining factor 1 and a different part determining factor 2.

Notation for new systems

It is possible that new factors in addition to those currently known will be discovered and shown to be inherited independently of any of the known systems. If this occurs it seems advisable to relate the system symbol to the immunoglobulins and to the appropriate polypeptide chain and to rename the currently established Gm and Inv systems so that their symbols reflect the structural units they control. In this event, it is suggested that the symbol " I " be used as the initial letter in the description of all the loci for the immunoglobulins.

Notation for new factors

There is no wish to restrict the freedom of investigators to publish data in any way they desire. On the other hand, the usefulness of the proposed system of notation will be seriously jeopardized if numerical symbols are added to the present list in an uncoordinated way. For these reasons, the following recommendations are made:

(*a*) If the serological and family data are insufficient to meet the criteria for recognition of new factors set out below, either because of insufficient quantity of the reagent or because the frequency of the factor in the population precludes definitive family studies, it is recommended that the author give the new factor a provisional name using a two-letter abbreviation derived from town name, name of patient, etc. This should be preceded by the non-specific generic term I, rather than a specific system symbol, e.g., I(pr) and I(−pr) for the phenotypes.

(*b*) If the factor which has not yet been assigned a number is known to be part of the Gm or Inv systems, it can be indicated in the parenthesis after the numbered factors, for example: Gm(1,−2,3,4, 5,pr) or Gm(1,3,4,5,pr).

(*c*) If the author believes that the criteria are fulfilled and that the linkage relations have been established, the use of a number instead of the provisional name is warranted. To avoid duplicate use of the same number a request for a number should be sent to the WHO International Reference Centre for Genetic Factors of Human Immunoglobulins, addressed to Dr C. Ropartz, Directeur, Centre départemental de Transfusion sanguine et de Génétique humaine, 609, Chemin de la Bretèque, 76–Bois-Guillaume, France.

(*d*) If the factor is shown to belong to one of the already known linkage groups (systems), it would be assigned the next available number of that group, e.g., Inv(4).

(*e*) If the factor is shown to belong to a different system, it would be given the number 1. If it is located on a particular immunoglobulin class, the system symbol could be chosen according to the suggestions made above. In choosing the system symbol for a factor not localized on one particular class of immunoglobulins, transposition of the provisional letter into the system symbol might be useful. The phenotype I(pr) would in this instance be changed to IPr(1).

None of these suggestions should be taken to imply any formal control over the future use of numbers to describe factors inherited in the immunoglobulins. The sole intention is to avoid duplication of numbers or their use for poorly defined factors, and to assist in the rapid inclusion of reported factors into the proposed system of notation. Circulation of data relevant to their identification to other investigators would be helpful in this respect.

Criteria for recognition of new factors

To establish that a test system detects a " new " factor, it is recommended that the following conditions be fulfilled:

(*a*) The reaction system employed should show complete reproducibility. With the current haemagglutination-inhibition technique, the difference between " inhibiting " and " non-inhibiting " normal sera from the same population should be three tubes or higher in a twofold dilution test system.

(*b*) Since antisera may contain mixtures of antibodies of different specificities, steps should be taken to show that the observed " new " reaction patterns are not due to an obvious mixture of antibodies of previously known specificities. (Absorption experiments using cells coated with selected antibodies, inhibition tests with purified myeloma proteins, and tests for consistency using cells coated with antibodies from different persons may give information concerning these matters.)

(*c*) It is essential to specify all reagents used in any study because,

(1) two reagents (antiglobulin and a cell coat) are necessary to define a factor;

(2) the same coated cells in some cases may be used for defining more than one factor; and

(3) the antiglobulin from one person may be used with different cell coats to define more than one factor. For example:

Factor	*Anti-globulin*	*Dilution*	*Cell coat*	*Dilution*
Gm(5)	Dr.*	1/8	Anti-D V.S.*	1/5
Gm(13)	Th.*	1/8	Anti-D V.S.*	1/5
Gm(6)	Bomb.*	1/32	Anti-D Warren *	1/10
Gm(5)	Bomb.*	1/32	Anti-D Berg *	1/10

* Identification of reagent.

(*d*) Enough family data should be obtained to establish the pattern of inheritance of the new factor.

(*e*) Tests with isolated immunoglobulins from positive and negative sera should be performed to show that the new factor is associated with immunoglobulins. Tests with agammaglobulinaemic sera might also be useful.

(*f*) The reactions observed with the new set of reagents should be different in at least one race from those of any previously described set of reagents. It is suggested that a useful standard for deciding that the new factor differs from known factors is a χ^2 test of the comparisons of the reaction with different reagent sets, giving values with a $P \leqslant 0.02$. However, one clearly established and inherited difference, confirmed in several laboratories, may be acceptable as evidence for a new factor.

Reference panel of sera

In order to maintain uniformity in reagent sets used to detect established differences between the immunoglobulins of different individuals,the specificities of the reagent sets should be defined by their reactions with a reference panel of normal human sera. It is hoped that such a panel will be made available through the WHO International Reference Centre for Genetic Factors of Human Immunoglobulins.

* * *

R. Ceppellini, Institute of Medical Genetics, University of Turin, Turin, Italy
S. Dray, Department of Microbiology, University of Illinois, Chicago, Ill., U.S.A.
J. L. Fahey, National Cancer Institute, National Institutes of Health, Bethesda, Md, USA
E. C. Franklin, Department of Medicine, New York University School of Medicine, New York, N.Y., USA
H. Fudenberg, Department of Medicine, University of California, San Francisco Medical Center, San Francisco, Calif., USA
P. G. H. Gell, Department of Experimental Pathology, School of Medicine, University of Birmingham, Birmingham, England
H. C. Goodman, Immunology, World Health Organization, Geneva, Switzerland
R. Grubb, Institute of Bacteriology, Lund, Sweden
M. Harboe, Institutt for Eksperimentell Medisinsk Forskning, Oslo, Norway
R. L. Kirk, Human Genetics, World Health Organization, Geneva, Switzerland
J. Oudin, Institut Pasteur, Paris, France
C. Ropartz, Centre départemental de Transfusion sanguine et de Génétique humaine, 76–Bois-Guillaume, France
O. Smithies, Department of Medical Genetics, University of Wisconsin, Madison, Wis., USA
A. G. Steinberg, Western Reserve University, Cleveland, Ohio, USA
Z. Trnka, Immunology, World Health Organization, Geneva, Switzerland

NOTATION FOR HUMAN IMMUNOGLOBULIN SUBCLASSES *

After consultation between immunologists from a number of countries a nomenclature for human immunoglobulins was proposed in 1964 and was published in the Bulletin of the World Health Organization.[1] *However, that proposed scheme of notation, which has already gained wide acceptance, left several specialized areas of nomenclature still to be resolved; one of these was the subclasses of immunoglobulins. Some of the research workers most closely concerned with the problem have now agreed upon a unified scheme for the notation of the human immunoglobulin subclasses, and, in particular, of the immunoglobulin G subclass, for which two different nomenclatorial schemes have been followed in recent years. Their proposals are given below.*

Human immunoglobulin molecules can be divided into at least four major groups or classes, referred to either as IgG, IgA, IgM and IgD, or as γG, γA, γM and γD, as suggested in 1964.[1]

Recent studies in many laboratories have shown that several of these classes can be further divided into subclasses, and consequently, several temporary subclass designations have come into use.

Considerable information has been obtained concerning immunoglobulin G and A subclasses, and it now seems appropriate (1) to put forward a uniform notation for the immunoglobulin G subclasses, and (2) to propose a general scheme for the notation of additional immunoglobulin subclasses as they are described.

The general proposal is as follows:

(1) Subclasses should be indicated by an arabic numeral following the letter denoting the class. Arabic rather than Roman numerals are suggested because of their greater simplicity. Confusion with the genetic factors can be avoided by listing genetic factors in parentheses, preferably preceded by the locus.

(2) Subclasses should be numbered on the basis of relative concentration in normal serum or on the basis of relative frequency of occurrence as myeloma proteins.

(3) When potential new subclasses are first identified, the investigator should employ a temporary designation in accordance with the nomenclature proposed in 1964[1] (initial, city, etc.), but this designation should not resemble the numerical terminology herein proposed.

(4) Final numerical subclass notations should be used only when several laboratories have exchanged reagents and agreed on the categorization.

The specific proposal for IgG (γG) is shown below:

Current	*Occurrence as myeloma proteins (%)*	*Proposed*	*Polypeptide heavy chain (γ-chain)*
We or γ2b or C	70-80	IgG1 or γG1	γ1
Ne or γ2a	13-18	IgG2 or γG2	γ2
Vi or γ2c or Z	6-8	IgG3 or γG3	γ3
Ge or γ2d	3	IgG4 or γG4	γ4

Thus a type K myeloma protein currently classed as Vi, Z-type or γ2c would be called IgG3-K or γG3-K; and the heavy chain would be designated γ3.

It is hoped that the proposed scheme will prove a useful aid in communicating current information about human immunoglobulin subclasses while retaining flexibility for designating new subclasses in the future.

* A French version will be published in a later issue.
[1] *Bull. Wld Hlth Org.*, 1964, **30**, 447-450.

* * *

HENRY G. KUNKEL, Rockefeller University, New York, N.Y., USA.
JOHN L. FAHEY, National Cancer Institute, National Institutes of Health, Bethesda, Md., USA.
EDWARD C. FRANKLIN, Department of Medicine, New York University School of Medicine, New York, N.Y., USA.
ELLIOTT F. OSSERMAN, Department of Medicine, College of Physicians and Surgeons of Columbia University, New York, N.Y., USA.
WILLIAM D. TERRY, National Cancer Institute, National Institutes of Health, Bethesda, Md., USA.

ADDENDUM

The three subclasses of human immunoglobulin designated as γA, γB and γC by S. Dray correspond to subclasses γG2, γG1 and γG3, respectively, in the proposed notation.

IMMUNOGLOBULIN E, A NEW CLASS OF HUMAN IMMUNOGLOBULIN *

Studies of the nature of the antibodies associated with isologous skin-sensitizing activity have indicated the presence of a previously unrecognized immunoglobulin in human serum. The immunoglobulin has been identified by virtue of specific antigenic determinants. Independently, a protein with similar antigen characteristics has been identified both in the serum of a patient with multiple myeloma and in normal serum. It is proposed that the normal protein and antigenically related myeloma proteins shall be designated IgE or γE, and the heavy polypeptide chains of these molecules be designated ϵ (epsilon)-chains, in accordance with an earlier memorandum entitled *Nomenclature for Human Immunoglobulins.*[a] This replaces the previous usage of γE-globulin and IgND.

IgE has antigenic determinants in common with other immunoglobulin classes, as well as specific antigenic determinants. IgE from non-myeloma sources has been found to contain the determinants of light chains of Type K and Type L. The E myeloma protein has been found to have light chains of Type L. The specific antigenic determinants of IgE have not been detected in IgG, IgA, IgM and IgD. Antisera specific for IgE have failed to react with immunoglobulins of these four classes and their currently recognized subclasses. Conversely antisera specific for these classes and their subclasses have failed to react with IgE.

Studies on the E myeloma protein have shown that it contains heavy and light polypeptide chains with respective molecular weights of approximately 75 500 and 22 500. The unique determinants of IgE were not present on its light chains. The IgE determinants have not yet been directly demonstrated on the isolated heavy chains, but are thought to be located there for the following reasons.

(*a*) Digestion of the E myeloma protein with papain produced two kinds of fragments, referred to as Fab- and Fc-fragments by analogy with the fragments produced by the action of papain on IgG. The Fab-fragment contained light chain determinants but no IgE determinants. The Fc-fragment lacked light chain determinants. The IgE specific determinants were found only on this fragment.

(*b*) Molecular weight data were consistent with the Fc-fragment being a portion of the heavy chains. The molecular weight of the intact molecule was found to be approximately 200 000. Following complete reduction and dissociation, 20% of the protein was recovered as light chains of molecular weight of approximately 22 500, indicating two light chains per molecule. Assuming two heavy chains per molecule the molecular weight of each heavy chain was calculated to be approximately 75 500. The Fc-fragment had an approximate molecular weight of 100 000, as estimated from sedimentation and gel-filtration data.

Consideration of the antigenic analysis and the physicochemical data has therefore indicated that IgE determinants are located in the heavy chains of the molecule.

There is evidence for antibody activity in IgE. IgE from selected sera has been shown to combine with a number of antigens in several techniques of radioimmunoassay. The specificity of these reactions is comparable to the specificity of antigen-binding by other classes of immunoglobulins.

In studies of immediate-type hypersensitivity the binding activity of IgE for a given allergen in various human sera was found to correlate with the ability

* This memorandum was drafted by the signatories (see overleaf) following discussions held at the WHO International Reference Centre for Immunoglobulins in Lausanne in February 1968. A French version will be published in a later issue.

[a] *Bull. Wld Hlth Org.*, 1964, **30**, 447-450.

of these sera passively to sensitize human skin to that allergen. IgE non-reactive with specific allergen and the E myeloma protein blocked this sensitization. The ability to induce or block isologous passive skin sensitization may be a characteristic of the human IgE class.

* * *

H. H. Bennich, Institute of Biochemistry, University of Uppsala, Uppsala, Sweden
K. Ishizaka, Children's Asthma Research Institute and Hospital, Denver, Colo., USA
S. G. O. Johansson, Blood Centre, University Hospital, Uppsala, Sweden
D. S. Rowe, Director, WHO International Reference Centre for Immunoglobulins, Institut de Biochimie, Lausanne, Switzerland
D. R. Stanworth, Department of Experimental Pathology, University of Birmingham, Birmingham, England
W. D. Terry, National Cancer Institute, National Institutes of Health, Bethesda, Md., USA

AN EXTENSION OF THE NOMENCLATURE FOR IMMUNOGLOBULINS *

Earlier proposals for the nomenclature of human immunoglobulins [1] have been generally accepted. Recent studies of the remarkable heterogeneity of immunoglobulins and of antibodies have produced additional findings on human immunoglobulins which require the extension of the existing terminology. Certain new terms are therefore proposed for well-established properties of the structure and amino acid sequences of the heavy and light chains of these proteins. These additions to the terminology should help in defining those regions of antibody molecules which are responsible for their two major kinds of functions—i.e., the function of antigen binding and those other functions which are manifested by biological properties such as complement fixation.

Definition of the regions of immunoglobulin molecules

It is now clear that the polypeptide chains of immunoglobulins consist of 2 well-defined regions which are here designated " the variable region " and " the constant region ". The variable region has been so designated because of the diversity of its amino acid sequences, whereas the constant region is relatively invariable in molecules of the same class and type. It is recommended that the variable and constant regions be termed the " V region " and the " C region " respectively. It is proposed that the symbols " V_L " and " C_L " be generic terms for the variable and the constant regions of light chains and that " V_H" and " C_H" be generic terms for the corresponding regions of heavy chains. If it is desired to specify a particular class or subclass of heavy chain, the symbol " H " could be replaced by the symbol of the chain. For example, the C_H region of a heavy chain of a molecule of the IgG1 subclass would be designated " $C_{\gamma 1}$ region ". Similarly, if it is desired to specify a particular type of light chain, the symbol " L " could be replaced by the symbol for the chain: for example, " V_κ region ", $C\lambda$ region." [2]

The exact length of these regions cannot be specified. In human light chains the V_L and C_L regions have about the same number of amino acid residues. For example, in the κ (kappa) chains so far studied the VL regions consist of 107 to 113 residues beginning at the amino terminus and the CL regions consist of the remaining 107 residues. Heavy chains have been less extensively studied than have light chains. For γ (gamma) chains the available data on complete sequences of human heavy chains show that the V_H region is of approximately the same length as the V_L region of the same molecule and that the C_H region consists of 3 linearly arranged adjacent regions which show homologies with C_L and with each other. Less extensive data on other human gamma chains and on rabbit gamma chains suggest that this will be a general finding in chains of the gamma class. It is therefore proposed that such regions in γ1 heavy chains, for example, be named " homology region $C_{\gamma 1}1$ ", " homology region $C_{\gamma 1}2$ ", " homology region $C_{\gamma 1}3$ ", and so on, beginning with the homology region which is closest to the amino terminus of the chain. If similar homology regions are found in other classes, the appropriate chain symbol would be employed, e.g., " homology region $C_\alpha 1$ ", " homology region $C_\mu 1$ ", etc.

Nomenclature of half-cystinyl residues

It is suggested that half-cystinyl residues be designated by Roman numerals, the first residue being that which is closest to the amino terminus. An Arabic numeral (to be placed as a subscript) corresponds to the number of the amino acid residue in the chain being described. This will satisfactorily permit the representation of intrachain and interchain disulfide bonds as well as of free sulfhydryl groups. Intrachain bonds can be designated, for example, " disulfide bond κ (I_{23}–II_{88}) ". Interchain bonds can be designated as follows: " disulfide bond

---

* This memorandum was drafted by the signatories (see page 977) following discussions held during a WHO meeting on the nomenclature of immunoglobulins that took place on 9-11 June 1969 in Prague. A French version will be published in a later issue.

[1] *Bull. Wld Hlth Org.*, 1964, **30**, 447; 1965, **33**, 721; 1966, **35**, 953; 1968, **38**, 151.

[2] The symbol " L " has been suggested previously for the L type of immunoglobulins (*Bull. Wld Hlth Org.*, 1964, **30**, 447). The usage of the subscript " L ", as in " V_L " and " C_L " is distinct: subscript " L " specifies light chains irrespective of type.

κV_{214}–γIV_{200}" and " disulfide bond $\gamma 1 VI_{226}$–$\gamma 1 VI_{226}$". In all matters of chemical terminology the rules of IUPAC–IUB [1] should be observed.

Definition of groups and subgroups

All variable regions associated with a light chain of given type are defined as a " group ". Subdivisions may be distinguished within a group. These subdivisions are called " subgroups " and are designated by Roman numerals. In human κ-chain groups at least 3 discrete sets of sequences have been recognized. These are now called " subgroup $V_{\kappa I}$", " subgroup $V_{\kappa II}$" and " subgroup $V_{\kappa III}$". Similarly, in human λ (lambda) chains at least 5 sets of sequences have now been recognized: these are called " subgroup $V_{\lambda I}$", etc. The correspondence between the present usage and the proposed usage is shown in the accompanying table. The subgroups

LIGHT CHAIN SUBGROUPS

Light chain [a]	Present usage			Proposed usage
κ chains	$S_{\kappa I}$,	Tra,	Basic group I	$V_{\kappa I}$
	$S_{\kappa II}$,[b]	Smi,[b]	Basic group III	$V_{\kappa II}$
	$S_{\kappa II}$,[b]	Smi,[b]	Basic group II	$V_{\kappa III}$
λ chains	I,	$S_{\lambda II}$		$V_{\lambda I}$
	II,[b]	$S_{\lambda I}$		$V_{\lambda II}$
	IV,	other		$V_{\lambda III}$
	II,[b]	$S_{\lambda III}$		$V_{\lambda IV}$
	III,	other		$V_{\lambda V}$

[a] References:

κ chain:
Hood, L., Gray, W. R., Sanders, B. G. & Dreyer, W. J. (1967) *Cold Spr. Harb. Symp. quant. Biol.*, **32**, 133.
Niall, H. & Edman, P. (1967) *Nature (Lond.)*, **216**, 263.
Milstein, C. (1967) *Nature (Lond.)*, **216**, 330.

λ chain:
Langer, B., Steinmetz-Kayne, M. & Hilschmann, N. (1968) *Hoppe-Seylers Z. physiol Chem.*, **349**, 945.
Hood, L. & Ein, D. (1968) *Nature (Lond.)*, **220**, 764.

[b] These subgroups were not further separated at the time of publication.

have been designated I, II and III, etc. in order of their frequency of occurrence in the chains which have so far been studied. This follows the nomenclature of subclasses of heavy chains of IgG, which are also numbered in order of frequency of occurrence.[2] Prototype sequences of 20 residues of the subgroups beginning at the amino terminus are given in the Annex to this paper.

Definition of classes and subclasses and types and subtypes

C_H and C_L regions show heterogeneity. This is the basis of the recognition of classes of heavy chains and types of light chains. Subdivisions of classes have previously been designated subclasses. It is proposed that similar subdivisions of types be designated " subtypes " and that the principles for their nomenclature should be the same as those for subclasses. The terms " classes " and " subclasses ", " types " and " subtypes " specifically exclude differences arising owing to allelism.

Formulae for immunoglobulin molecules

The over-all structure of immunoglobulins may be represented by formulae. Thus, an IgG1 molecule with κ light chains of subgroup I could be written

$$[(V_{\kappa I}C_{\kappa})\ (V_{\gamma}C_{\gamma 1})]_2$$

If it is desired to include homology regions, this could be expanded to

$$[(V_{\kappa I}C_{\kappa})\ (V_{\gamma}\ C_{\gamma 1}1\ C_{\gamma 1}2\ C_{\gamma 1}3)]_2$$

Presence inside the square brackets indicates association of light and heavy chains, the formula for each of which is in parentheses. The subscript 2 outside the brackets indicates that the association of 2 such units forms the molecule. An IgM molecule with κ light chains may be represented, by use of the brace, as

$$\{[(V_{\kappa}C_{\kappa})\ (V_{\mu}C_{\mu})]_2\}_5$$

Formulae could be especially useful in representing certain γA immunoglobulins in which the 2 light chains are linked as $(V_{\kappa}C_{\kappa})_2$ and the heavy chains as $(V_{\alpha}C_{\alpha})_2$ to give

$$[(V_{\kappa}C_{\kappa})_2\ (V_{\alpha}C_{\alpha})_2]$$

Immunoglobulins of secretions

The IgA in the external secretions of man and several other species has a molecular structure characterized by the presence of an additional component which is lacking in IgA derived from serum. This additional component is sometimes encountered not bound to IgA. It is suggested that it be designated " secretory component " or " S

[1] See, for instance, IUPAC–IUB Commission on Biochemical Nomenclature (1966) *J. biol. Chem.*, **241**, 527, 2491.

[2] *Bull. Wld Hlth Org.*, 1966, **35**, 953.

component " and that other terms such as " transport piece " should not be used. The term " secretory " in the definition is not meant to imply any function but rather to indicate the characteristic association with secretions of IgA possessing this additional component.

* * *

R. Asofski, National Institute of Allergy and Infectious Diseases, Bethesda, Md., USA

R. A. Binaghi, Laboratoire de Médecine expérimentale, Collège de France, Paris, France

G. M. Edelman, The Rockefeller University, New York, N.Y., USA

H. C. Goodman, Immunology, World Health Organization, Geneva, Switzerland

J. F. Heremans, Cliniques universitaires St Pierre, Université catholique de Louvain, Louvain, Belgium

L. Hood, National Cancer Institute, Bethesda, Md., USA

E. A. Kabat, Columbia-Presbyterian Medical Center, New York, N.Y., USA

J. Rejnek, Department of Immunology, Institute of Microbiology, Prague, Czechoslovakia

D. S. Rowe, Director, WHO International Reference Centre for Immunoglobulins, Lausanne, Switzerland

P. A. Small, Jr, Department of Microbiology, College of Medicine, University of Florida, Gainsville, Fla., USA

Z. Trnka, Immunology, World Health Organization, Geneva, Switzerland

Annex

PROTOTYPE AMINO-TERMINUS SEQUENCES OF THE SUBGROUPS OF HUMAN κ AND λ LIGHT CHAINS [a]

Sub-groups	Sequence
	κ chains
$V_{\kappa}I$	Asp – Ile – Gln – Met – Thr – Gln – Ser – Pro – Ser – Ser – Leu – Ser – Ala – Ser – Val – Gly – Asp – Arg – Val – Thr
$V_{\kappa}II$	Glu – Ile – Val – Leu – Thr – Gln – Ser – Pro – Gly – Thr – Leu – Ser – Leu – Ser – Pro – Gly – Glu – Arg – Ala – Thr
$V_{\kappa}III$	Asp – Ile – Val – Met – Thr – Gln – Ser – Pro – Leu – Ser – Leu – Pro – Val – Thr – Pro – Gly – Glu – Pro – Ala – Ser
	λ chains
$V_{\lambda}I$	Glp – Ser – Val – Leu – Thr – Gln – Pro – Pro – [ ] – Ser – Val – Ser – Gly – Ala – Pro – Gly – Gln – Arg – Val – Thr
$V_{\lambda}II$	Glp – Ser – Ala – Leu – Thr – Gln – Pro – Ala – [ ] – Ser – Val – Ser – Gly – Ser – Pro – Gly – Gln – Ser – Ile – Thr
$V_{\lambda}III$	[ ] – Tyr – Val – Leu – Thr – Gln – Pro – Pro – [ ] – Ser – Val – Ser – Val – Ser – Pro – Gly – Gln – Thr – Ala – Ser
$V_{\lambda}IV$	Glp – Ser – Ala – Leu – Thr – Gln – Pro – Pro – [ ] – Ser – Ala – Ser – Gly – Ser – Pro – Gly – Gln – Ser – Val – Thr
$V_{\lambda}V$	[ ] – Ser – Glu – Leu – Thr – Gln – Pro – Pro – [ ] – Ala – Val – Ser – Val – Ala – Leu – Gly – Gln – Thr – Val – Arg

[a] The symbol Glp indicates the residue derived from pyrrolid-2-one-5-carboxylic acid.

Nomenclature of human immunoglobulins

The Nomenclature Committee of the International Union of Immunological Societies recently approved the following amendments [1] to the nomenclature for human immunoglobulins that was recommended in 1964. [2]

1. All immunoglobulins should be designated by the letters Ig; the Greek letter gamma (γ) should no longer be used for this purpose, but should be used solely to designate the heavy polypeptide chains of immunoglobulin G (IgG). (The use of the term "gamma-globulin" to designate immunoglobulins is therefore not permissible.) Examples:

Present usage	*Recommended usage*
γG1 or IgG1	IgG1
γD or IgD	IgD

2. The letter L should be used only to designate light polypeptide chains (heavy chains being designated by the letter H), and should no longer be used to designate molecules whose light chains are of the lambda type. Molecules or isolated light chains of this type should be designated "lambda type" or "λ type". Example:

Present usage	*Recommended usage*
IgML	IgM(λ)

3. The letter K, which has been used to designate molecules whose light polypeptide chains are of the kappa type, should no longer be used. Molecules or isolated light chains of this type should be designated "kappa type" or "κ type". Example:

Present usage	*Recommended usage*
IgGK	IgG(κ)

4. No changes are made in the previous proposals [3] for the terms class, subclass, type, subtype, group, and subgroup. However, the proposals for the nomenclature of subgroups are at present under revision and will be the subject of future recommendations.

---

[1] *Biochemistry* (1972), **11**, 3311.
[2] *Bull. Wld Hlth Org.*, **30**, 447.
[3] *Bull. Wld Hlth Org.* (1964), **30**, 447; (1969), **41**, 975.

Proposed rules for the designation of immunoglobulins of animal origin *

The present article sets forth proposed rules for the designation of immunoglobulins of animal origin and their chains. It also recommends symbols to be used for the designation of classes and types, subclasses and subtypes, (sub)subclasses and (sub)subtypes, and allotypes. Recommended rules for the designation of newly discovered polypeptide chains are also included.

Various nomenclatures are in use to designate immunoglobulins of animal origin. In order to avoid confusion, the Nomenclature Subcommittee for Animal Immunoglobulins of the IUIS felt that rules for the designation of these immunoglobulins and their chains should be established, and that these rules should follow as far as possible similar rules established for the designation of human immunoglobulins.[a, b]

SYMBOLS FOR IMMUNOGLOBULIN (Ig) MOLECULES AND THEIR HEAVY (H) AND LIGHT (L) POLYPEPTIDE CHAINS

Distinction between Ig and H-chain symbols

The previous recommendation [b] relating to human immunoglobulins that the use of the symbol γ be restricted to the designation of a particular class of H chains is reiterated and emphasized for immunoglobulins of animal origin. Terms such as "γ-globulin" or "γ G" should not be used. The correct term in the example cited is IgG.

Structure of the L- and H-chain symbols

In their complete form these symbols (referring to the constant regions of L or H chains) contain three structural elements designating (*a*) *the category of chain* (L-chain type or H-chain class), (*b*) *isotypic rank* (e.g., subclass), and (*c*) *allotype* of the chains involved.

The allotypic term is added only when required. The isotypic rank item is indicated only when distinctions such as subtype or subclass are known to occur within the type of L chain or class of H chain in question.

CHAIN CATEGORY SYMBOLS

The *category* symbol or *chain* symbol is the main component of the name of an Ig polypeptide chain. It always consists of a single, small Greek letter.

The symbols used for the different L-chain types characterized so far are κ (kappa) and λ (lambda).

* These proposed rules on the designation of immunoglobulins of animal origin were prepared by the Nomenclature Subcommittee for Animal Immunoglobulins of the International Union of Immunological Societies (IUIS). The members of the Subcommittee are listed on page 817. A French translation of this Terminology Note will appear in a future issue of the *Bulletin*.

[a] *Biochemistry*, **11**: 331 (1972).

[b] *Bulletin of the World Health Organization*, **48**: 373 (1973).

The symbols used for the different L-chain classes characterized so far are γ (gamma), μ (mu), α (alpha), δ (delta) and ε (epsilon).

The symbol of a newly-characterized animal Ig polypeptide chain should, where possible, be the same as that already used for other polypeptide chains to which the new chain has been demonstrated to be structurally related. In the absence of such information, the rules for provisional symbols (see below) will apply.

ISOTYPIC RANK SYMBOLS

Definition of classes and types, subclasses and subtypes, and (sub)subclasses and (sub)subtypes

Classes of H chains and *types* of L chains are defined as isotypic categories (C-region variants coded for by separate loci) of these chains, showing large differences in their constant regions. Within a given species, antigenic relationships between the C regions of H chains of different classes, or of L chains of different types cannot, as a rule, be demonstrated.

The first level of subdivision of classes is into subclasses. C_H regions of a given subclass possess certain antigenic or primary structural features characteristic of, and exclusive to, the subclass and other features common to all C_H regions of the class.

In some cases, a second level of subdivision into (sub)subclasses may be necessary. C_H regions of a given (sub)subclass possess certain features characteristic of, and exclusive to, the (sub)subclass and other features common to all C_H regions of the subclass and class.

Light-chain types may similarly be divided into subtypes and (sub)subtypes.

Evolutionary divergence of the C regions of classes and types appears to have proceeded independently in different species or groups of species. Therefore, the subdivisions recognized in one species may have no counterparts in other species and their nomenclature is not necessarily based on homology. In addition, the prefixes sub and (sub) represent only a ranking order of diversity within a given class or type of a species; they carry no implication of the degree of divergence.

In the case of a newly characterized chain in which structural homology with some already described chain(s) appears possible or probable, the name should be chosen accordingly to avoid later changes.

Symbols for subclasses and subtypes and for (sub)subclasses and (sub)subtypes

The part of the name of a chain that specifies its rank within a class or type should be written as a postscript to the class or type symbol of the chain that is specified.

Subclasses of H chains and *subtypes* of L chains are always indicated by an Arabic numeral.

(Sub)subclasses of H chains and, if required, *(sub)subtypes* of L chains are always indicated by a small Latin letter, which is always written after the subclass or subtype numeral, for example:

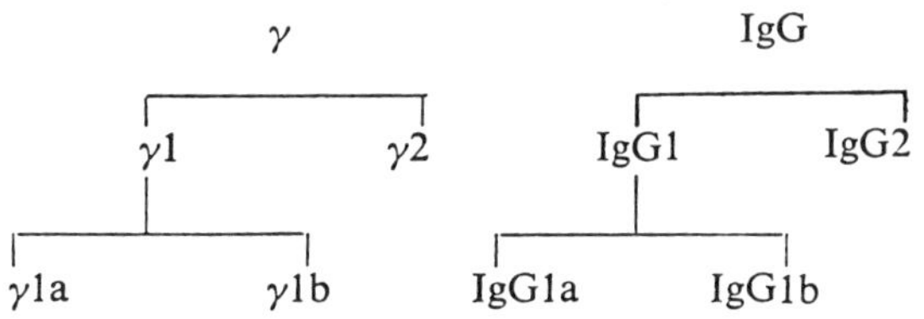

Chains Corresponding Ig molecules

ALLOTYPIC SYMBOLS

The symbol for the allotype of the chain, if such exists and is required, should be placed in parentheses *after* the chain symbol and on the same level as the latter.

NAMES FOR IMMUNOGLOBULIN MOLECULES

In compliance with previous recommendations, the name of an Ig molecule always begins with the symbol Ig, followed by the Latin capital equivalent of a small Greek letter indicating the name of the H chain.

PROVISIONAL SYMBOLS

Rules for chain symbols

(*a*) Should the newly described Ig polypeptide chain be firmly identified as corresponding to the same class or type as other already named Ig polypeptide chains, the name of the latter should be used for it.

(*b*) Should such identification be only tentative, the name of the supposedly related chain should be written within single quotation marks.

(*c*) Only if the newly described chain demonstrably constitutes a class or type not yet named in the literature should a novel chain symbol be proposed for it. In the case of H chains, this symbol should be a Greek letter having a Latin equivalent from which a name for the corresponding Ig can be derived.

(*d*) In the absence of sufficient information in certain non-mammalian species, a provisional name with descriptive connotations (e.g., 7.4 S Ig) should be used.

Examples:

Novel chain	*Novel Ig*
(*a*) γ	IgG
(*b*) 'γ'	Ig 'G'
(*c*) β	IgB
(*d*) H chain of 7.4 S Ig	7.4 S Ig

Rules for isotypic rank symbols

Where chain symbols appear within single quotation marks, the isotypic rank symbol should also be included in these, for example:

Ig 'G2'
'α2' chains

* * *

H. Ambrosius, Karl-Marx University, Leipzig, German Democratic Republic.

R. Asofsky, National Institutes of Health, Bethesda, MD, USA.

R. A. Binaghi, Collège de France, Paris, France.

D. Capra, University of Texas, Southwestern Medical School, Dallas, TX, USA.

L. Hood, California Institute of Technology, Pasadena, CA, USA.

E. Orlans, Chester Beatty Research Institute, Sutton, Surrey, England.

D. S. Rowe, World Health Organization, Geneva, Switzerland.

P. Small, University of Florida, College of Medicine, Gainesville, FL, USA.

G. Torrigiani, World Health Organization, Geneva, Switzerland.

J.-P. Vaerman, Institute of Cellular Pathology, University of Louvain, Brussels, Belgium.

Nomenclature for synthetic peptides representative of immunoglobulin chain sequences*

WHO–IUIS Nomenclature Sub-Committee[1]

The source (species of origin), type, and subgroup (where applicable) of the immunoglobulin chain are indicated prior to the numbers of the first and last amino acid residues comprising the synthesized sequence (stated in parentheses), e.g., human γ_1 (289–298) or rat ε (143–147).

Square brackets indicate that the peptide is an analogue; substituted amino acids are identified by the three-letter code; superscripted numbers indicating the residue at which the substitution, removal or addition occurs. Further substitutions are specified within round brackets. For example, human γ_1 (289–298) [D-Thr^{298}] and human γ_1 (289–298) [Asn (CHO)^{297}].

Background

Current interest in immunologically active peptides is by no means confined to analogues of thymic hormones or complement components; nor to those short-chain peptides which have been shown to possess granulocyte chemotactic activity. In recent years, there has been growing interest in the application of protein synthesis as an alternative strategy to proteolytic and chemical fragmentation in the location and characterization of immunoglobulins (as discussed, for instance, by Stanworth (*16*)). Furthermore, this is leading, in many cases, to the development of potentially therapeutic peptides with important immunomodulatory properties. The forerunner of these developments was the synthesis of tuftsin (Thr-Lys-Pro-Arg), representative of a tetrapeptide sequence within the C_H2 domains of human IgG (*13*), which was shown to possess phagocytosis-stimulating activity.

Since then, short-chain linear peptides with sequences representative of other putative immunoglobulin Fc effector sites have been synthesized and studied; for instance, peptides capable of inhibiting the binding by IgG of C1q (*1,10*), the binding of IgG to Fc receptors on monocytes and macrophages (*3, 14*), and the action of IgG antibody in ADCC (antibody-dependent cellular cytotoxicity) (*5*) and NK (natural killer cell) activity (*6*).

The synthetic peptide approach has also been exploited extensively in attempts to identify both mast cell Fc receptor-binding sites (*7,17*) and trigger sites (*16, 17*). More recently, antibodies raised against peptides have been used as IgE structural probes (e.g., Burt et al. (*2*)); and immunoglobulin peptides produced by DNA recombinant technology have been employed in similar types of investigation (e.g., Helm et al. (*8*), Duncan & Winter (*4*)). Furthermore, synthetic peptides representative of both C_H2 and C_H3 domain sequences within human IgG have been shown to provide a direct activating signal to resting human B lymphocytes and to enhance antibody production *in vitro* and *in vivo* (*15*), as well as to induce immunoglobulin synthesis by murine B cells (*9, 12*).

It is against this background that it is considered timely to establish a nomenclature for synthetic peptides representative of imunoglobulin heavy and light chain sequences that is acceptable to investigators working in this field and which will facilitate communication and discussion. In the preparation of the following peptide nomenclature proposals, it was considered most important (in view of the tendency

*This article was drafted by a group of experts working under the auspices of the International Union of Immunological Societies (IUIS) and has been approved by the Nomenclature Committee of the IUIS. Members of the group were D.R. Stanworth (*Chairman*), K.J. Dorrington, T.E. Hugli, K. Reid and M.W. Turner. A French translation appears on pages 112–114. Requests for reprints and all correspondence should be addressed to the Chairman of the IUIS Nomenclature Committee, Dr M.D. Kazatchkine, Unité d'Immunopathologie, Hôpital Broussais, 96 rue Didot, 75014 Paris, France.

Reprint No. **5052**

of different laboratories to use a different immunoglobulin amino acid numbering system) to refer to a standard source for information about the detailed primary structures of immunoglobulin polypeptide chains; it is suggested that this source should be *Sequences of proteins of immunological interest* edited by Elvin A. Kabat and colleagues. The 4th edition was published by the U.S. Elvin A. Kabat and colleagues. The 4th edition was published by the U.S. Department of Health and Human Services in 1987.

Nomenclature for synthetic peptides

Human immunoglobulin heavy or light chain sequences

Where a peptide has been assigned a name, e.g., tuftsin (comprising residues 289–301 of the human γ_1 chain) or rigin (comprising residues 345–349 of the same chain), it would be expected that it would be referred to in this way in the rest of an article. Otherwise, it is suggested that a nomenclature be adopted which is consistent with that applied to other types of peptide, e.g., hormones. Thus, the source, type and subgroup (where applicable) of the immunoglobulin chain will be indicated prior to the numbers of the first and last amino acid residues comprising the synthesized sequence (stated in parentheses), e.g., human γ_1 (289–298), rat ε (143–147), and human K_{II}[pGlú-6].

It will be important to indicate the species of origin and the subclass of heavy chain; but it should not be necessary to specify the domain, provided that the complete numbered sequence of the chain in question has been reported in the literature (to which reference would presumably be made in any publication in which the peptide is referred to). If this is not the case, it will be necessary to specify the full primary sequence of the synthesized peptide, preferably using the three letter code (unless lack of space dictates otherwise). Indeed, at an appropriate position in any publication (e.g., as a table or footnote), it would be expected to provide the full peptide sequences alongside the nomenclatures which have been assigned to them.

It is customary now to specify the numbers of the amino acids comprising the synthesized sequence on the line and in parentheses; rather than below, as a subscript (as was the practice in referring to peptide hormones, etc. in the past).

Analogues

It is important to specify when synthetic peptides are *derivatives* of sequences contained within the native immunoglobulin polypeptide chain structure. Thus the use of [ ] indicates that the peptide referred to is an *analogue*; and the substitutions or modifications in the analogue are indicated as to type (the amino acid identified by three-letter code). The use of ( ) within the square brackets specifies further substitution; whilst superscripted number(s) indicate the residue at which the substitution, removal or addition occurs. Obviously, where there have been several substitutions (or derivatizations) of particular residues in the parent peptide it will not be feasible to give anything but the full modified sequence. But, where such changes have been minimal, an abbreviated nomenclature would be useful. Examples of these are:

human γ_1 (289–298) [D-Thr^{298}]
human γ_1 (289–298) [Asn^{297}]
human γ_1 (289–298) [Gly $(NH_2)^{298}$]
human γ_1 (289–298) [Glu^{293}, Lys^{297}]
human γ_1 (289–298) [Asn$(CHO)^{297}$].

As indicated in the third example above, and in one of the examples given in the previous section, it is necessary to indicate whether the COOH-terminal carboxyl or the NH_2-terminal α-amino group has been derivatized.

Allotypic differences can be identified in the same manner as substitutions, provided that the reference sequence is understood or there is agreement as to the original form. For example:

human γ_3 (289–298) [Thr^{296}]—referring to the G3m(g) allotype
human γ_3 (289–298) [Phe^{296}]—referring to the nG3m(g) allotype.

Proteolytic and chemical cleavage fragments

It is assumed that the currently accepted nomenclature referring to cleavage fragments of immunoglobulins (for example, Fc, Fab, Fc′, $F(ab')_2$, Facb, pFc′, tFc′, TLmFc, etc.) will continue to be used, in which case it is suggested that such products are referred to as *fragments* rather than as peptides, as has sometimes been the practice (e.g., Morgan et al. (*11*)).

References

1. **Boackle, R.J. et al.** An IgG primary sequence theory for complement activation using synthetic peptides. *Nature*, **282**: 742–743 (1980).
2. **Burt, D.S. et al.** Analysis of the interaction between rat immunoglobulin E and rat mast cells using anti-peptide antibodies. *Molecular immunology*, **24**: 379–389 (1987).
3. **Ciccimara, F. et al.** Localisation of the IgG effector site for monocyte receptors. *Proceedings of the National Academy of Sciences of the USA*, **72**: 2081–2083 (1975).

4. **Duncan, A.R. & Winter, G.** The binding site for C1q on IgG. *Nature*, **332**: 738–740 (1988).
5. **Gergely, J. et al.** Binding characteristics and isotype specificity of Fc receptors in K cells. *Molecular immunology*. **23**: 1203–1209 (1986).
6. **Gherman, M. et al.** Regulation of human natural cytotoxicity by IgG. 1. Characterisation of the structural site on monomeric IgG responsible for inhibiting natural killer cell activity. *Molecular immunology*, **24**: 743–750 (1987).
7. **Hamburger, R.N.** Peptide inhibition of Prausnitz–Küstner reaction. *Science*, **189**: 389–390 (1975).
8. **Helm, B. et al.** The mast cell binding site on human immunoglobulin E. *Nature*, **331**: 180–183 (1988).
9. **Hobbs, M.V. et al.** Fc peptide mediated regulation of the immune response. II. Analysis of secreted immunoglobulin classes, accessory cell contribution and lymphocyte proliferation in p23 stimulated spleen cell cultures. *Journal of immunology*, **134**: 2847–2852 (1985).
10. **Lukas, T.J. et al.** Inhibition of C1-mediated immune haemolysis by monomeric and dimeric peptides from the second constant domain of human immunoglobulin G. *Journal of immunology*, **127**: 2555–2560 (1981).
11. **Morgan, E.L. et al.** Isolation and identification of a biologically active peptide derived from the C_H3 domain of human IgG1. *Proceedings of the National Academy of Sciences of the USA*, **79**: 5388–5391 (1982).
12. **Morgan, E.L. et al.** Synthetic Fc peptide mediated regulation of the immune response. 1. Characterisation of the immunomodulatory properties of a synthetic 23 amino acid peptide derived from the sequence of the C_H3 domain of IgG1. *Journal of experimental medicine* **157**: 944–947 (1983).
13. **Najjar, V.A. & Nishioka, K.** Tuftsin—a physiological phagocytosis-stimulating peptide. *Nature*, **228**: 672–673 (1970).
14. **Ratcliffe, A. & Stanworth, D.R.** The use of synthetic γ-chain peptides in the localisation of the binding site(s) on human IgG1 for the Fc receptors of homologous monocytes and heterologous mouse macrophages. *Immunology letters*, **4**: 215–221 (1982).
15. **Sármay, G. et al.** The effect of synthetic peptides corresponding to Fc sequences in human IgG1 on various steps on the B cell activation pathway. *European journal of immunology*, **18**: 289–294 (1988).
16. **Stanworth, D.R.** Application of synthetic peptides representative of immunoglobulin sequences to the delineation of receptor binding and signalling processes. *Molecular immunology*, **19**: 1245–1254 (1982).
17. **Stanworth, D.R. et al.** *The use of synthetic peptides in the delineation of immunoglobulin antigenic epitopes and Fc effector functions.* Ciba Foundation Symposium 119, 1986, pp. 226–244.

Nomenclature of immunoglobulin A and other proteins of the mucosal immune system*

IUIS/WHO Subcommittee on IgA Nomenclature[1]

The predominant immunoglobulin found in exocrine secretions of humans and most other mammals is secretory IgA, a polymeric form of IgA containing an additional glycoprotein chain designated "secretory component". In this article recommended abbreviations are proposed for the following forms of human IgA and other proteins of related interest: secretory IgA, secretory IgM, secretory component, polymeric immunoglobulin receptor, polymeric IgA, monomeric IgA, IgA subclass 1, IgA subclass 2, A2 allotype marker 1, and A2 allotype marker 2.

Background and definitions

The predominant immunoglobulin found in exocrine secretions of humans and most other mammals is secretory IgA, a polymeric form of IgA containing an additional glycoprotein chain, designated "secretory component". Secretory IgM, a form of IgM containing bound secretory component, also occurs in secretions, and elevated levels may be present in IgA-deficient humans. Secretory component is synthesized in epithelial and glandular cells, in which it is first expressed as a basolateral membrane receptor for J-chain-containing polymeric immunoglobulins, and has therefore been referred to as "polymeric immunoglobulin receptor". During transepithelial transport in endocytic vesicles, polymeric IgA usually becomes covalently linked through formation of disulfide bonds to the secretory component, which is proteolytically cleaved from its transmembrane segment before exocytotic release of the complete secretory IgA at the apical surface. IgM is similarly transported to form secretory IgM, except that disulfide bonds are not formed with secretory component. The circulatory form of IgA does not contain secretory component, but may occur in both monomeric and J-chain-containing polymeric forms. Although various abbreviations for secretory IgA are in common use, none has been formally recognized by the IUIS/WHO Nomenclature Committee. Confusion arises because of the frequent usage of the abbreviation "sIg" for surface immunoglobulin (with isotype designations as appropriate) on B lymphocytes.

In humans, two subclasses of IgA are known (IgA1 and IgA2), and similar subclasses have been identified in certain other primates (gorilla, chimpanzee, and gibbon). Most other mammals (and other vertebrates in which IgA has been found) have no currently known subclasses of IgA, with the notable exception of the Lagomorpha (rabbits and their allies), which have 13 subclasses. In addition, human IgA2 exhibits allotypic polymorphism; at least two allotypes that have been defined serologically and at the molecular level are widely distributed in the human gene pool. Additional forms of IgA2 have been described, but it is not clear whether they all represent true allelic variants. Previous reports of the IUIS/WHO Nomenclature Committee have defined subclasses and allotypes of IgG (*1*, *2*), but no formal nomenclature exists for the subclasses and allotypes of IgA.

Nomenclature

The recommendations (see Table 1) are based upon previously approved nomenclature for

---

* Drafted by the Nomenclature Committee of the Society for Mucosal Immunology (SMI), following approval of the proposals by the Board and Membership of SMI at the Ninth International Congress of Mucosal Immunology, Sydney, Australia, 27–31 January 1997. This report has been approved by the IUIS/WHO Nomenclature Committee. A résumé in French appears on page 428.

Requests for reprints should be addressed to the Chairman of the IUIS Nomenclature Committee, Professor M.W. Turner, Immunobiology Unit, Institute of Child Health, 30 Guilford Street, London WC1N 1EH, England.

[1] M.W. Russell (*Chairman*) and M. Gleeson. *Co-signatories*: P. Brandtzaeg, A. Ferguson, L.Å. Hanson, M.E. Lamm, J. Mestecky, I. Moro, B.J. Underdown, and J.-P. Vaerman.

Reprint No. **5879**

Table 1: **Recommended abbreviations for various forms of human IgA and other proteins of related interest**

S-IgA	Secretory IgA
S-IgM	Secretory IgM
SC	Secretory component
pIgR	Polymeric immunoglobulin receptor (membrane secretory component)
pIgA	Polymeric IgA
mIgA	Monomeric IgA
IgA1	IgA subclass 1
IgA2	IgA subclass 2
A2m(1)	A2 allotype marker 1
A2m(2)	A2 allotype marker 2

immunoglobulins, and extend the same principles to the designation of IgA subclasses and allotypes.

S-IgA and S-IgM are approved as abbreviations for secretory IgA and secretory IgM, respectively, to avoid confusion with surface immunoglobulins on B cells; accordingly, it is recommended that sIg be used to refer to surface immunoglobulins. S also relates to "SC" as the abbreviation for secretory component, which is the distinctive feature of S-IgA (and S-IgM). A significant minority has expressed the view that the hyphenated forms (S-IgA and S-IgM) are unnecessary, and may choose to use unhyphenated forms (SIgA and SIgM). The occasional practice of abbreviating serum IgA is disapproved as both unnecessary and confusing. The membrane form of secretory component, often referred to as polymeric immunoglobulin receptor, may be abbreviated as pIgR in conformity with other receptor nomenclature and existing practice. Polymeric IgA, which must normally contain J-chain to be so designated, may be abbreviated as pIgA, and monomeric IgA as mIgA. Although multiple forms of polymeric IgA exist (dimers, trimers, tetramers, and higher forms), it is infrequently necessary to make these distinctions, and accordingly it is undesirable to recommend standard abbreviations for them.

IgA subclass and allotype nomenclature is consistent with existing nomenclature for IgG subclasses and allotypes. IgA2 molecules carrying the allotypic markers may be referred to as IgA2m(1) or IgA2m(2). If additional allotypes of human IgA2 are confirmed, their designation should follow the same convention.

Where appropriate, these abbreviations, and the conventions on which they are based, should apply to the corresponding proteins of other animal species as well as the human proteins.

Résumé

Nomenclature des immunoglobulines A et autres protéines impliquées dans le système immunitaire mucosal

L'immunoglobuline la plus abondante des sécrétions exocrines de la plupart des mammifères et de l'homme est l'IgA sécrétoire, une forme polymérique d'IgA associée à une chaîne glycoprotéique appelée composant sécrétoire ou «pièce sécrétoire». On propose dans le présent article des abréviations recommandées pour les IgA humaines et les protéines apparentées suivantes: IgA sécrétoire, IgM sécrétoire, pièce sécrétoire, récepteur d'immunoglobuline polymérique, IgA polymérique, IgA monomérique, IgA sous-classe 1, IgA sous-classe 2, A2 marqueur allotypique 1, A2 marqueur allotypique 2.

References

1. Notation for genetic factors of human immunoglobulins. *Bulletin of the World Health Organization*, 1965, **33**: 721–724.
2. Notation for human immunoglobulin subclasses. *Bulletin of the World Health Organization*, 1966, **35**: 953.

Nomenclature for T-cell receptor (TCR) gene segments of the immune system*

WHO-IUIS Nomenclature Sub-Committee on TCR Designation[1]

The recommended procedures and criteria for T-cell receptor (TCR) designations are described. The officially adopted designations are for the TCR A, B, D and G loci and for V, D, J and C segments.

Principles of TCR nomenclature

The following principles and criteria should be observed.

(1) The intention is to develop a simple set of rules that can be applied to all TCR V, D, J and C loci and which are consistent with current trends in gene mapping nomenclature.

(2) The nomenclature should be applicable to all species and to systems characterized at any level from the first sequence to full mapping.

(3) To satisfy (2), the official name should not contain detailed information about gene order, pseudogenes, cDNA or genomic sequence, and the productive or non-productive nature of polymorphisms. Such additional information should be in parentheses after the official name.

(4) Gene segments should be named only when a full cDNA or genomic sequence is available. Naming is at the level of gene segments but data from the cDNA sequence may be used since for most genes only the cDNA sequence is available. A name for the rearranged gene product should be assembled from the loci names (see page 114, TCRD).

(5) The locus names (A, B, G, D) and genetic elements (V, D, J, C) are self-explanatory. S refers to gene segments and is used to enumerate and distinguish subfamily members. The TCR A and D V-segments present a problem since the same V region can be used for A or D TCR chains. In the present proposal one set of names is given for all A and D V-genes; the term A or D or both can be used in the name depending on whether the context is for TCR alpha or delta chains. Thus one might use TCRAV1S1 or TCRDV1S1 or TCRADV1S1 for the same V-gene in different contexts. This may seem unorthodox but once the A/D rule is known there is no problem since there will never be two A/D V-genes with the same V-S- name. The numbering of the few V-genes used *mainly or exclusively* in delta TCRs begin with 101, i.e., V101S1, V102S1, etc., allowing identification of unique delta families.

(6) An asterisk (*) will separate alleles from loci, consistent with gene mapping rules.

Nomenclature of human TCR gene segments

The officially adopted designations for TCRA, TCRB, TCRG, TCRD (no hyphen separates TCR from A, B, G or D) loci are described below.

(1) *TCRA*

TCRAV1S1 TCRAV1S2 TCRAV1S3	Distinct loci but these members are of the same family, where S refers to family member. See note 1 (Annex).
TCRAV2S1	Second family.
TCRADV1S1	When the V region can be used by alpha or delta, A, D or AD can be used. See principle 5 (above).
TCRAV1S1*1 TCRAV1S1*2	Alleles at the same locus. See notes 2 to 8 (Annex).

---

* This article was drafted by a group of experts working under the auspices of the International Union of Immunological Societies (IUIS) and has been approved by the Nomenclature Committee of IUIS. Requests for reprints and all correspondence should be addressed to the Chairman of the IUIS Nomenclature Committee, Professor Michel Kazatchkine, Unite d'Immunologie, Hôpital Broussais, 96 rue Didot, 75014 Paris, France. A French translation of this Terminology Note will appear in a later issue of the *Bulletin*.

[1] Members of the Nomenclature Sub-Committee: A.F. Williams (United Kingdom) (*Chairman*), J.L. Strominger (USA) (*Co-Chairman*), and J. Bell (United Kingdom) (*Co-Chairman*), T.W. Mak (Canada), J. Kappler (USA), P. Marrack (USA), B. Arden (Germany), M.P. Lefranc (France), L. Hood (USA), S. Toneqawa (USA), and M. Davis (USA). Standing Committee on TCR Designation: T.W. Mak (*Chairman*), Ontario Cancer Institute, Princess Margaret Hospital, Toronto, Ontario, Canada, and B. Arden, Paul Ehrlich Institute, Langen, Germany.

Reprint No. **5362**

TCRAJ1S1 S2	To designate J region families and their members.
TCRAC1	
*1 *2	To designate AC locus. For AC alleles if found.

Further description, when available, could be provided in parentheses. See note 5 (Annex).

(2) *TCRB*

TCRBV1S1 BV1S2 BV2S1	Exactly as for TCRAV.
*1 *2 *3	If alleles are found.
TCRBD1 TCRBD2	For the 2 D loci.
*1 *2	If alleles are found.
TCRBJ1S1 TCRBJ1S2 TCRBJ1S3 TCRBJ2S1 TCRBJ2S2 TCRBJ2S3	For the J region loci. See note 9 (Annex).
*1 *2	If alleles are found.
TCRBC1 TCRBC2	For the two BC loci

(3) *TCRG*

TCRGV1S1 S2	For the V family with multiple segments.
TCRGV2S1	For all of the other segments including pseudogenes. See note 4 (Annex).
*1 *2	To be added if alleles are found.
TCRGJ1S1 TCRGJ1S2 TCRGJ1S3 TCRGJ2S1	
*1 *2	To be added if alleles are found.
TCRGC1	
GC2*1 *2 *3	For alleles of the 2nd GC segment.

(4) *TCRD*

TCRDV101S1	As for the AV segments or with the 101 etc. names. See principle 5 (above).
TCRADV101S1	Where the sequence used in both alpha and delta AD can be used.
TCRDV101S2	
*1 *2	To be added if alleles are found.
TCRDD1 TCRDD2 TCRDD3	For the D region genomic segments.
*1 *2	See note 10 (Annex).
TCRDJ1S1 TCRDJ1S2 TCRDJ2S1	For the 3 J segments.
*1 *2	For alleles as before.
TCRDC1	For the only DC segment.

Name for a rearranged gene product

A complete name for a rearranged TCRA gene (for example) could be:

TCRAV1S1J1S2C1.

Various shorthand versions could be used within a paper after the first complete naming:

V1S1J1S2C1
or V1S1J1S2
or VA1S1J1S2
or VA1S1
or VA1.1
or VB2S2J1S2 (for a TCRB gene)
or VB2S2
or VB2.2

i.e., in a paper this last abbreviation would describe TCRBV2S2J1S2C1 (thereafter called VB2S2 or VB2.2).

Annex

Notes

(1) Criteria for distribution to families have been given detailed consideration and will be included in a forthcoming publication.

(2) Alleles should only be named if it is certain they are true alleles. If it is possible that they are pseudoalleles (product of a distinct locus), then they should be initially named as a family member but product of a distinct locus, e.g., AV1S1, AV1S2, AV1S3, etc. When proven to be truly allelic, the designation can be changed, e.g., AV1S3 could be changed to AV1S1*2 if it were allelic to AV1S1*1. Alleles are defined at the nucleic acid level.

(3) Care must be taken to *avoid* using N addition nucleotides to designate a V, D or J segment as an allele.

(4) If two identical sequences exist at different loci, these could bear the same name but be distinguished by a or b after the name, i.e. TCRAV1S1*1a or TCRAV1S1*1b.

(5) At the end of the official nomenclature a parenthesis after the official name would contain information about:

(a)	gene order	(23)
(b)	pseudogenes	(P)
(c)	orphon genes	(O)
(d)	nonproductive substitutions	(N)
(e)	tentative designation	(T)

(5a) The gene order would require complete genomic mapping of a complex and would also address duplicate genes.

(5b) Pseudogenes may be shown as a P after the official name. P would only be used when the sequence indicating a functional TCR could not be formed using this segment (e.g., frame shift from a single base deletion, stop codon, loss of an essential amino acid, etc.); i.e., TCRAV1S3*1P.

(5c) For example, a processed pseudogene. Similarly, additional information about loci mapping outside the complex could be denoted by the letter O (orphon).

(5d) An allelic nucleotide substitution that does not result in an amino acid change.

(5e) When an incomplete sequence is obtained and clearly represents a new gene segment, it can be designated as tentative (T). This designation can be removed when the sequence is completed.
For example:

	TCRAV1S1*1(43, P)	Representing in order the locus number from the C region, in this case a pseudogene.
or	TCRAV1S1*2(43, N)	In this case a nonproductive allelic variant.
or	TCRAV1S7(O)	An orphon gene.

(6) Where the allelic polymorphism is the deletion of a gene, this could be designated by V1S1*O.

(7) In order to be assigned a name, the sequence would have to be referenced (published or in press). Once the nomenclature is introduced and accepted, then all new sequences should be submitted to the Standing Committee by authors and/or editors for naming prior to publication (as is now done in the HLA field).

(8) It would be difficult to insist that a cell line be deposited and available for verification (as is done for HLA alleles) because many TCR sequences are derived from factor-dependent lines (some easily lost) by PCR (polymerase chain reaction), etc. There does not seem to be an easy way to deal with this problem.

(9) The J region loci are classed according to genomic localization, not sequence similarity. This is the one exception with the rest of the nomenclature.

(10) Where multiple D segments are used in the transcript, this can be expressed as follows:

TCRDV1S2D2D3J2C1.

NOMENCLATURE FOR FACTORS OF THE HL-A SYSTEM *

At the Third Conference on Histocompatibility Testing, held at Saint-Vincent, Italy, in July 1967, the participants agreed to appoint, by postal vote, a Nomenclature Committee drawn from among specialists in tissue typing, immunology and human genetics; that Committee was asked to propose a nomenclature for leucocyte antigens, which, it was hoped, might prove internationally acceptable. The Secretariat of the World Health Organization was asked to facilitate and assist in the work of the Committee. The following is the text of the memorandum drawn up by the Committee.[1]

After description of the first human leucocyte iso-antigen, Mac, in 1958, several other leucocyte and platelet specificities were defined by agglutination, complement-fixation and cytotoxicity techniques. These factors were found on a variety of tissue cells and the possibility that they were histocompatibility antigens was proposed. Definition of antigenic specificities and of genetic relationships among them was greatly facilitated by the introduction of computer analysis. Many leucocyte and platelet factors have now been detected. The intricate relationships among them, evident from population and linkage studies, led to the concept that most of these specificities belonged to a single complex system. This was confirmed by family studies combining serology, skin grafting, and lymphocyte-culture techniques. An international nomenclature committee proposed that the major locus be designated HL-A.[2] The present report concerns the nomenclature of well-recognized specificities within the HL-A system. It does not relate to other antigenic systems.

Until now, most of the specificities defined by anti-leucocyte antibodies have been given different names by various laboratories. In devising a new nomenclature, the Nomenclature Committee attempted to use numbers which coincided, whenever possible, with those already in most common use, without regard to priorities or supposed genetic relationships.

Unanimous agreement was reached on naming certain specificities for which evidence had been obtained during histocompatibility-testing workshops and by exchange of sera (see the table).

Description of nomenclature

The use of subscripts, italics, lower-case letters, and similar devices was avoided for ease in composition, communication and computation.

The Committee recommended that a distinct specificity should be designated by number. Closely related but slightly different specificities should be distinguished by the addition of a figure after a full point. Specificities designated by a given number will have a high positive correlation coefficient, generally greater than 0.90. To establish that two closely related specificities are different, the discordant reactions must be shown to be reproducible. Identification of the donor of the antibody and the date of bleeding are considered to be an essential part of the description and designation of a serum in all reports.

A series of serological factors, such as the HL-A specificities, are grouped into a system if the recombination fractions between their corresponding genetic determinants are small. The effective limit on these recombination fractions is set by the resolution

* A French version will be published in a later issue.

[1] The members of the Committee were: Dr F. H. ALLEN, New York Blood Center, New York, N.Y., USA; Professor D. B. AMOS, Duke Medical Center, Durham, N.C., USA (*Chairman*); Dr J. R. BATCHELOR, Queen Victoria Hospital, East Grinstead, Sussex, England; Dr W. F. BODMER, Stanford University School of Medicine, Palo Alto, Calif., USA; Professor R. CEPPELLINI, Institute of Medical Genetics, University of Turin, Turin, Italy; Professor J. DAUSSET, Institut de Recherches sur les Maladies du Sang, Hôpital St-Louis, Paris, France; Dr R. D. OWEN, California Institute of Technology, Pasadena, Calif., USA (*Vice-Chairman*); Dr ROSE PAYNE, Stanford University School of Medicine, Palo Alto, Calif., USA; Dr J. J. VAN ROOD, University of Leiden, Leiden, Netherlands; Dr N. R. SHULMAN, National Institute of Arthritis and Metabolic Diseases, Bethesda, Md., USA; Dr P. I. TERASAKI, University of California School of Medicine, Los Angeles, Calif., USA; Dr Z. TRNKA, Immunology, World Health Organization, Geneva, Switzerland (*Acting Secretary*); Dr R. L. WALFORD, University of California School of Medicine, Los Angeles, Calif., USA.

[2] Amos, D. B. (1968) *Science*, **160**, 659-660.

NEW HL-A NOMENCLATURE AND PREVIOUS DESIGNATIONS [a]

New HL-A nomenclature [b]	Amos	Batchelor	Ceppellini	Dausset	Kissmeyer-Nielsen	Payne/Bodmer	van Rood	Shulman	Terasaki	Walford
HL-A1	19	1	To-8	11	LA1	LA1	LA1	—	1	Lc-1
HL-A2, or HL-AMac	1	5	To-9	1 or Mac	LA2	LA2	8a	PlGrLy^{B1}	2	Lc-2
HL-A3	4	—	To-10	12	LA3	LA3	LA3	Hill	8	Lc-3
HL-A4										
HL-A5	45	25	To-5	5	—	—	Da5	—	6	—
HL-A6										
HL-A7	2	—	To-20	10	—	4d	7c	—	5	Lc-8
HL-A8	41	2	To-7	8	—	7d	7d	—	11	Lc-7

[a] A dash (—) indicates that no symbol has been allocated within the nomenclature concerned.

[b] HL-A4 will be reserved for one of the higher frequency 4[a] factors, and HL-A6 for 4[b]. Before assigning these specificities, an exchange of serum among collaborating laboratories will be necessary.

of human pedigree studies and so is unlikely to be much less than 1%. A frequent, but not necessary, consequence of such close linkage is association among the factors at the population level. This association may vary from one population to another. The recognition of a new factor belonging to a system, such as HL-A, depends, therefore, not only on a population correlation analysis with established HL-A factors but also on family studies. The families studied must be directly informative with respect to recombination involving the postulated new factor. The Committee recommends that, in order to be assigned to the HL-A system, a new factor should show no recombination among a total of at least 20 genetically informative children from at least 3 families. This makes independence between the new factor and the HL-A system unlikely, though it does not exclude comparatively loose linkage—for example, with a recombination fraction of about 10% at a probability level of 0.1. Further family studies showing recombination between HL-A factors at a level below 1%, or chemical evidence leading to an understanding of gene–antigen relationships may, in the future, justify subdivision of the HL-A system into smaller genetic units. The assignment to such a subdivision would then be indicated by a common symbol immediately preceding the numbers defining the subunit factors.

Notational system

In the presentation of the data the factors typed for and the typing reagents should be specified. Serological factors are indicated by the number following the symbol for the system, e.g., HL-A1, HL-A2, etc. Other factors having a high positive correlation with a primary factor are indicated by a second number following a full point, e.g., HL-A2 for the original factor and HL-A2.1 for the associated factor.

An individual's complex phenotype may be presented in a table reporting the serological reactions. In the text the phenotype should be represented by the system symbol followed by the numbers corresponding to the factors which were found to be positive, these being separated by commas. For example, a donor who is positive with factors 1, 2, 7, and 8 and negative with 3 would be designated HL-A1,2,7,8. To make this meaningful, the antisera used must be listed, so that *negative* reactions may be known even though they are not indicated directly in the statement of the phenotype.

The genotype must be derived from family segregation analysis that identifies the two sets of factors controlled by the two homologous chromosomes. These sets, or haplotypes, are indicated within parentheses by the factors that are inherited in coupling; thus, for the example given above, the haplotypes could be HL-A(1,8) and HL-A(2,7). The genotype is indicated by the two haplotypes separated by an oblique stroke (solidus), for example, HL-A(1,8/2,7).

Allocation of numbers

The following procedures are recommended for obtaining international designations for HL-A factors. Until certification is obtained, a local designation [1] is appropriate; numbers preceded by the symbols HL-A should not be used.

Preliminary testing in laboratory of origin. The investigator should screen sera suspected of defining new specificities on his own cell panel, comparing them with antisera defining known HL-A specificities. The following steps are recommended:

1. The investigator should attempt to obtain more than one serum defining the supposed new specificity.

2. The reagents should be available in quantities of at least 200 ml. (Smaller quantities of high-titred serum could be considered equivalent.)

3. The reagents should give a reproducibility of at least 95% by a recognized technique designated by the investigator.

4. They should be mono- or oligospecific on the basis of absorptions with at least 10 positive cells when retested on the immunizing donor or on at least 10 highly reactive cells.

Certification.

1. The sera should be tested on members of 3 or more genetically informative families containing at least 20 children and should show no recombination with HL-A factors.

2. When these criteria have been fulfilled, the evidence should be submitted to a WHO collaborating laboratory. The laboratory may make available to the investigator cells, fresh or frozen, from its own panel of characterized donors. Details of the procedure will be agreed upon by the investigator and the laboratory involved.

3. Ultimately, the reagent must be shown to be operationally monospecific by absorption with, in general, cells from not fewer than 30 positive subjects if the frequency of reaction is greater than 15%, or from 15 positive donors if the frequency is less than 15%.

4. If the specificity is confirmed as apparently new, verification should be obtained from a second collaborating laboratory.

5. All relevant data will be submitted to the Acting Secretary of this Nomenclature Committee, who will circularize collaborating laboratories for a postal vote.

6. The Acting Secretary will then allocate a designation, if the specificity does not correspond to any previously designated factor.

Two sera can be considered to define the same specificity only if they give identical results when tested on a panel containing approximately 100 cells, of which at least 10 should be positively reacting and 10 negative. Any discrepancies that exist on first testing should disappear on repeated testing or following absorption.

* * *

Laboratories that have consented to act on a voluntary basis as WHO collaborating laboratories for leucocyte antigens are those of:

Dr D. B. Amos and C. Zmijewski, Department of Microbiology and Immunology, Duke Medical Center, Durham, N.C., USA.

Dr J. R. Batchelor, McIndoe Memorial Research Unit, Blond Laboratories, Queen Victoria Hospital, East Grinstead, Sussex, England

Professor R. Ceppellini, Institute of Medical Genetics, University of Turin, Turin, Italy

Professor J. Dausset, Institut de Recherches sur les Maladies du Sang, Hôpital St-Louis, 2 Place du Docteur-Fournier, Paris X^e^, France

Dr P. Ivanyi, Institute of Experimental Biology and Genetics, Czechoslovak Academy of Sciences, Budejovicka 1083, Prague 4, Czechoslovakia

Dr F. Kissmeyer-Nielsen, Blood Bank and Blood Grouping Laboratory, Aarhus Community Hospital, Aarhus, Denmark

Dr P. J. Morris, Department of Surgery, University of Melbourne, Parkville N.2., Melbourne, Australia

[1] See: Curtoni, E. S., Mattiuz, P. L. & Tosi, R. M., ed. (1967) *Histocompatibility testing 1967; Report of a Conference and Workshop, Torino and Saint-Vincent, Italy, 14-24 June 1967*, Copenhagen, Munksgaard.

Dr Rose Payne and Dr W. Bodmer, Department of Medicine (Haematology), Stanford University School of Medicine, Palo Alto, Calif. 94304, USA

Dr J. J. van Rood, Department of Immunohaematology, University of Leiden, Leiden, Netherlands

Dr N. R. Shulman, Clinical Haematology Branch, National Institute of Arthritis and Metabolic Diseases, National Institutes of Health, Bethesda, Md. 20014, USA

Dr P. I. Terasaki, Department of Surgery, School of Medicine, University of California, Los Angeles, Calif. 90024, USA

Dr R. A. Walford, School of Medicine, University of California, Los Angeles, Calif. 90024, USA

Dr C. van de Weerdt, Dr C. P. Engelfriet and Dr J. J. van Loghem, Central Laboratory of the Netherlands Red Cross Blood Transfusion Service, Plesmanlaan 125, Amsterdam, Netherlands

Nomenclature for factors of the HL–A system*

After the Third Conference on Histocompatibility Testing, a Nomenclature Committee drawn from among specialists in tissue typing, immunology, and human genetics proposed a nomenclature for leucocyte antigens, which has become accepted internationally. The text of the memorandum drawn up by the Committee was published in the Bulletin of the World Health Organization *(1968,* **39**, *483–486). After the Fifth Workshop on Histocompatibility, the Nomenclature Committee*[1] *decided that it was necessary to revise the 1968 memorandum. The following is the text of the revised memorandum.*

Since the first human leucocyte isoantigens were described in the late 1950s, the number of leucocyte and platelet specificities defined by agglutination, complement fixation, and cytotoxicity techniques has been increasing. These factors are found on a variety of tissue cells and the possibility that they are histocompatibility antigens has been proposed. The definition of antigenic specificities and of genetic relationships among them was greatly facilitated by the introduction of computer analysis. Many leucocyte and platelet factors have been detected. The intricate relationships among them, evident from population and linkage studies, has led to the concept that most of these specificities belong to a single complex system. In this system, the specificities can be arranged in two segregant series and, within each series, each specificity behaves as if determined by one of a mutually exclusive set of alleles.

This major system was designated HL-A. The relevance of HL-A as an immunogenetic marker was confirmed by family studies combining serology, skin grafting, and lymphocyte culture techniques. The present memorandum concerns the nomenclature of specificities within the HL-A system and does not relate to other antigenic systems.

The definition of a histocompatibility antigen of the HL-A system passes through four stages. In the first, a new specificity is detected by a laboratory and given that laboratory's designation. Next, if this specificity is confirmed by several of the reference laboratories (see the Annex) it is given a provisional number preceded by the prefix W. In the third stage, when firm agreement has been reached by all the reference laboratories on the definition of this new specificity, an HL-A number can be designated. Finally, the fourth stage, which has not yet been reached, would allow the chemical confirmation of this HL-A specificity.

Since 1968, a number of specificities have been given HL-A numbers. The following ones remain relatively well defined: HL-A1, HL-A2, HL-A3, HL-A7, HL-A8, HL-A11, HL-A12, and HL-A13. Problems have arisen with HL-A9, which appears to represent a cross reactivity between two components, HL-A10 and HL-A5. The latter also seem to be associated with a number of cross-reacting specificities that are still difficult to disentangle in non-caucasoid populations.

Description of nomenclature

The use of subscripts, italics, lower-case letters, and similar devices is avoided for ease of composition, communication, and computation. In the 1968 memorandum[1] the Committee recommended that a distinct specificity should be designated by a number and that closely related but different specificities should be indicated by adding a figure after a full stop. However, the Committee has now decided that this notation should be abandoned as it implies a biological relationship between factors, which may not be correct. In future a new specificity that is part of a broader HL-A specificity will be given a new number by the Committee. The designation will be reported initially as a W specificity. For example, the two components of HL-A9 will now be designated W23 and W24 (Table 1), but HL-A9 will continue to be defined as the broader specificity. The assignment of W numbers that do not overlap with existing HL-A numbers allows for the possibility

* A French version will be published in a later issue of the *Bulletin*.

[1] See list of signatories on pages 661-662.

Table 1. New HL-A designations and representative equivalents

New designations	Representative equivalents
W16	U18, Da31 (included in U18), Ge12, Sa533, Te64, Ao81
W21	Da24, ET, ?M3, ?Te61
W23	HL-A9.1, Da27 (9′), Lc-12
W24	HL-A9.2, Da32 (9″), BIM
W25	HL-A10.1, To31, Da29 (10″)
W26	HL-A10.2, To40, Da28 (10′)
W29	W19.1, Ao77, Bt15, Da22, Ge33, Te63
W30	W19.3, Da25′ (Da26), Lc-21, Te66
W31	W19.4, LAW, Da25′ (Da33), Lc-26.1
W32	W19.5, Ao28, To30, Ge32, Te59

that, when an antigen to which a W number has been provisionally assigned becomes eligible for an HL-A number, it can keep the same number. Table 1 shows the specificities to which W numbers have been assigned and their equivalent terms. These assignments arose out of the Fifth International Histocompatibility Workshop. At present it is not possible to state to what degree these newer factors are important in matching donors and recipients of organ transplants. It seems likely that the definition of families of cross-reacting specificities will be important in this respect, but knowledge of the components of these cross-reacting groups is still incomplete.

The HL-A phenotype of an individual will be represented by the system symbol followed by the numbers corresponding to the defined factors, separated by a comma—e.g., HL-A1, 2, 7, 8. Where one of the factors has a W designation, the phenotype will be expressed as before, but the W prefix will appear before the factor—e.g., HL-A1, W23, 7, W16.

The genotype must be derived from family segregation analysis (or another means of genetic analysis) that identifies the two sets of factors controlled by the two homologous chromosomes. These sets, or haplotypes, are indicated by the factors that are inherited in coupling, separated by a comma. Thus, for the examples given above, the haplotypes could be HL-A1, 8 and HL-A2, 7, and HL-A1, W16 and HL-A, W23, 7, respectively. The genotype is indicated by the two haplotypes separated by an oblique stroke (solidus)—e.g., HL-A, 8/2, 7.

A series of serological factors, such as the HL-A specificities, are grouped into a system if the recombination fractions between their corresponding genetic determinants are small. The effective limit on these recombination fractions is set by the resolution of human pedigree studies and so is unlikely to be much less than 1%. A frequent, but not inevitable, consequence of such close linkage is association among the factors at the population level. Such association may vary from one population to another. The recognition of a new factor belonging to a system such as HL-A depends, therefore, not only on a population correlation analysis with established HL-A factors, but also on family studies. The families studied must be directly informative with respect to recombination involving the postulated new factor. The Committee recommended that, in order to be assigned to the HL-A system, a new factor should show no recombination among a total of at least 20 genetically informative children from at least 3 families. This makes interdependence between the new factor and the HL-A system unlikely, although it does not exclude comparatively loose linkage—for example, with a recombination fraction of about 10% at a probability level of 0.1. Further family studies showing recombination between HL-A factors at a level below 1%, or chemical evidence leading to an understanding of gene–antigen relationships, may justify subdividing the HL-A system into small genetic units in future.

Allocation of numbers

The following procedures are recommended for obtaining international designations for HL-A factors. Until certification is obtained, a local designation is appropriate; numbers preceded by the symbols HL-A or W should not be used.

Preliminary testing in laboratory of origin. The investigator should screen, on his own cell panel, sera suspected of defining new specificities, comparing them with antisera defining known HL-A specificities. In addition, panels including individuals from different race groups can be very helpful and their use where appropriate is recommended. The following steps are recommended:

1. The investigator should attempt to obtain more than one serum defining the supposed new specificity.

2. The reagents should be available in quantities of at least 200 ml. (Smaller quantities of high-titred

[1] *Bull. Wld Hlth Org.*, 1968, **39**, 483-486.

serum may contain an equivalent amount of antibody.)

3. The reagents should give a reproducibility of at least 95% by a recognized technique designated by the investigator.

4. They should be monospecific or oligospecific on the basis of absorptions with at least 10 selected positive cells when retested on the immunizing donor or on at least 10 highly reactive cells. The use of cells that are known to have a blank allele of the appropriate series, as well as of cells that are known to be homozygous, will provide a more precise definition of a new specificity.

Certification

1. The sera should be tested on members of 3 or more genetically informative families containing at least 20 children and should show no recombination with HL-A factors.

2. When these criteria have been fulfilled, the evidence should be submitted to a WHO collaborating laboratory. The laboratory may supply the investigator with cells, fresh or frozen, from its own panel of characterized donors. Details of the procedure will be agreed upon by the investigator and the laboratory concerned.

3. Ultimately, the reagent must be shown to be operationally monospecific by absorption with, in general, cells from not fewer than 30 positive subjects if the frequency of reaction is greater than 15%, or from not fewer than 15 positive donors if the frequency is less than 15%.

4. If the specificity is confirmed as apparently new, verification should be obtained from a second collaborating laboratory.

5. All relevant data will then be considered by the Committee and, if the designation does not correspond to a previously designated factor, it will be given a W number.

Two sera can be considered to define the same specificity only if they give identical results when tested on a panel containing approximately 100 cells of which at least 10 should react positively and 10 negatively. Any discrepancies that exist on first testing should disappear on repeated testing or following absorption.

* * *

F. H. Allen, New York Blood Center, New York, N.Y., USA

D. B. Amos, Duke Medical Center, Durham, N.C., USA (*Chairman*)

J. R. Batchelor, Queen Victoria Hospital, East Grinstead, Sussex, England

W. F. Bodmer, University of Oxford, Oxford, England

R. Ceppellini, Institute of Medical Genetics, University of Turin, Italy

J. Dausset, Institut de Recherches sur les Maladies du Sang, Hôpital St-Louis, Paris, France

F. Kissmeyer-Nielsen, Aarhus Community Hospital, Aarhus, Denmark

P. J. Morris, University of Melbourne, Victoria, Australia (*Rapporteur*)

Rose Payne, Stanford University School of Medicine, Palo Alto, Calif., USA

J. J. van Rood, University of Leiden, Leiden, Netherlands

P. I. Terasaki, University of California School of Medicine, Los Angeles, Calif., USA

Z. Trnka, Basle Institute for Immunology, Basle, Switzerland (*Secretary*)

R. L. Walford, University of California School of Medicine, Los Angeles, Calif., USA

Annex

COLLABORATING LABORATORIES FOR LEUCOCYTE ANTIGEN TESTING

Professor D. B. Amos and Dr F. E. Ward, Department of Microbiology and Immunology, Duke University Medical Center, Durham, N.C., USA

Professor J. R. Batchelor, McIndoe Memorial Research Unit, Blond Laboratories, Queen Victoria Hospital, East Grinstead, Sussex, England

Professor W. F. Bodmer and Dr J. G. Bodmer, Genetics Laboratory, Department of Biochemistry, University of Oxford, Oxford, England

Professor R. Ceppellini, Centro Immunogenetica ed Istocompatibilità-CNR, c/o Institute of Medical Genetics, University of Turin, Turin, Italy

Professor J. Dausset and Dr J. Colombani, Institute for Research on Blood Diseases, Hôpital Saint-Louis, Paris, France

Dr P. Ivanyi, Institute of Experimental Biology and Genetics, Czechoslovak Academy of Sciences, Prague, Czechoslovakia

Dr M. Jeannet, Chief Medical Officer, Histocompatibility Laboratory, Geneva, Switzerland

Dr F. Kissmeyer-Nielsen, Blood Bank and Blood Grouping Laboratory, Aarhus Community Hospital, Aarhus, Denmark

Dr P. J. Morris, Tissue Transplantation Laboratories, Department of Surgery, University of Melbourne, The Royal Melbourne Hospital, Victoria, Australia

Dr Rose Payne, Dr C. Grumet, and Dr H. Perkins, Department of Medicine (Hematology), Stanford University School of Medicine, Palo Alto, Calif., USA

Dr J. J. van Rood, Department of Immunohaematology, University of Leiden, Leiden, Netherlands

Dr P. I. Terasaki, Department of Surgery, University of California School of Medicine, Los Angeles, Calif., USA

Dr R. L. Walford and Dr G. Smith, University of California School of Medicine, Los Angeles, Calif., USA

Dr C. P. Engelfriet and Dr J. J. van Loghem, Central Laboratory of the Netherlands Red Cross Blood Transfusion Service, Amsterdam, Netherlands

Nomenclature for factors of the HLA system, 1977 *

This article gives the decisions of the WHO nomenclature committee on leukocyte antigens, in particular concerning (a) the upgrading of certain HLA-A and HLA-B specificities to full HLA status, (b) the designation of new provisional specificities of the HLA-B, HLA-C, and HLA-D loci, and (c) the establishment of a nomenclature for the new specificities identified by serological techniques on B lymphocytes.

The WHO nomenclature committee on leukocyte antigens met under the auspices of the World Health Organization and the International Union of Immunological Societies, after the 7th Workshop on Histocompatibility Testing in Oxford in September 1977, with the aim of updating the nomenclature for specificities of the HLA-A, HLA-B, HLA-C, and HLA-D loci and establishing a nomenclature for the new specificities identified by serological techniques on B lymphocytes.

Previous reports in the *Bulletin of the World Health Organization* (*1*, *2*, *3*) have established a revised nomenclature for the HLA region. Taking into account advances in knowledge of the genetics of the major histocompatibility system of man it was agreed that HLA should be the name given to the whole region, while the terms HLA-A, HLA-B, HLA-C, and HLA-D should refer to the individual loci within it. Numbers following the locus symbols would identify individual specificities (e.g., HLA-A1), while the letter w following the locus symbol and preceding the number would indicate a provisionally identified specificity (e.g., HLA-Bw35).

The main aims of this report are:

(1) to upgrade certain HLA-A and HLA-B locus specificities to full HLA status.

(2) to designate new provisional specificities of the HLA-B, HLA-C and HLA-D loci.

(3) to establish a nomenclature for the new specificities identified by serological techniques on B lymphocytes.

Table 1. New designations for specificities of the HLA-A and HLA-B loci that have been upgraded to full HLA status

New	Previous
HLA-A25	HLA-Aw25
HLA-A26	HLA-Aw26
HLA-B15	HLA-Bw15
HLA-B17	HLA-Bw17
HLA-B37	HLA-Bw37
HLA-B40	HLA-Bw40

Specificities for HLA-A, HLA-B, and HLA-C loci

The newly upgraded specificities are listed in Table 1. In deciding which specificities should be upgraded, in addition to clarity and reproductibility of definition, general availability of the appropriate antisera was taken into account.

Although the specificities Cw1, Cw2, Cw3, and Cw4 are now considered to be sufficiently well defined to satisfy the qualifications for upgrading to full HLA status, it has been decided not to change the nomenclature, at least for the time being, to avoid any possible confusion with the nomenclature

* This terminology note was prepared by the WHO nomenclature committee on leukocyte antigens. The names of the members of the committee are listed on pages 464-465. The article has also been published in *Zeitschrift für Immunitätsforschung*, **153**: 373-379 (1977). A French version of this article will appear in a future issue of the *Bulletin*.

Table 2. New designations for provisional specificities of the HLA-B and HLA-C loci

New	Representative equivalents
HLA-Bw4	w4, 4a
HLA-Bw6	w6, 4b
HLA-Bw44	B12 (not TT *)
HLA-Bw45	TT *
HLA-Bw46	HS, SIN2
HLA-Bw47	407 *, MO66, CAS, Bw40C
HLA-Bw48	KSO, JA, Bw40.3
HLA-Bw49	Bw21.1, SL-ET
HLA-Bw50	Bw21.2, ET *
HLA-Bw51	B5.1
HLA-Bw52	B5.2
HLA-Bw53	HR
HLA-Bw54	Bw22j, SAP1
HLA-Cw6	T7

for the complement components C2 and C4, coded for, at least in part, by genes in the HLA region. Steps are being taken to consult with the IUIS Complement Nomenclature Sub-committee as to the symbols to be used for these complement loci.

New provisional designations for specificities of the HLA-B and HLA-C loci are listed in Table 2. These designations conform to the previously established principles—namely, that the specificities of the HLA-A and HLA-B loci are numbered jointly, so that there is no overlap in numbers between them, that numbers are retained for a specificity that may be split (e.g., HLA-A9, split into HLA-Aw23 and HLA-Aw24), and that numbers once used are never reassigned. It is recommended, however, that when both " broad " cross-reacting specificities and " narrow " or subtypic specificities are included in a phenotype designation, the broad specificities may be listed in parentheses at the end of the set of specificities for each locus, e.g., HLA-A1, 26 (10); B27, w50 (w21, w4, w6). The listing of broad specificities in this way, in addition to the narrow subtypic specificities, is optional. When, however, only the broad specificity is identified this is listed in the usual way, e.g., HLA-A1, 10; B27, w21.

HLA-Bw4 (previously w4 or 4a) and HLA-Bw6 (previously w6 or 4b) are now specifically associated with the B locus because of chemical evidence for their presence on the same molecules that carry the other HLA-B locus specificities. These two specificities often help considerably in distinguishing splits in B locus specificities. For example, in the case of HLA-Bw21 splits, HLA-Bw49 (previously Bw21.1 or SL-ET) is HLA-Bw4 associated while HLA-Bw50 (previously Bw21.2 or ET*) is HLA-Bw6 associated.

In certain cases, e.g., HLA-Bw53 (previously HR), a provisional specificity has been assigned even though all sera also contain antibodies against other specificities, in this case HLA-B5 and/or HLA-Bw35.

HLA-Bw45 (previously TT*) is most frequently found in certain African groups and is, for example, quite rare in European Caucasoid populations. This means that in practice, in European Caucasoids, HLA-B12 individuals are nearly always HLA-Bw44. When, however, sera identifying HLA-Bw45 have been used and an individual has been shown to be negative for this specificity, this person should be designated HLA-Bw44 or HLA-Bw44 (12) and not just HLA-B12.

In some cases it may be helpful to include a broad specificity in the genotype, following the same rules recommended above for the phenotype. For example, in the absence of sera identifying HLA-Bw45 but given typing for Bw4 and Bw6, a genotype HLA-A1, B8(w6)/A2, B12(w4) would clearly indicate that the HLA-A2, B12(w4) haplotype was probably HLA-A2, Bw44.

As is the case for a number of the previously established HLA specificities, certain of the newly designated provisional specificities are found predominantly in particular population groups, as already mentioned for Bw45. For example, HLA-Bw53 (previously HR) is found mainly in Negroes from Africa and America, HLA-Bw54 (previously Bw22J, etc.) and HLA-Bw46 (previously HS, SIN2) in Orientals and HLA-Bw48 (previously KSO, etc.) in Eskimos, American Indians, and possibly other oriental related populations.

The following suggested specificities were discussed, but were considered not yet sufficiently well defined to be assigned a provisional w designation: 9.3, 5.3, 5.4, 14.1, 14.2, 15.1, 15.2, 15A, 17 long, 17 short, 22.1, 22.2, DA30, 35A, 35C, 40.1, 40.2, DB, IM2, BU, T6.

HLA-D specificities

There has been a significant advance in the definition of certain of the HLA-D locus specificities, notably HLA-Dw1, HLA-Dw2, and HLA-Dw3. Nevertheless, the practical difficulties of cell typing do not yet justify the upgrading of any of these specificities to full HLA status. New designations for provisional specificities of the HLA-D locus are given in Table 3. The new specificity HLA-Dw11

Table 3. New designations for provisional specificities of the HLA-D locus

New	Previous or representative equivalent
HLA-Dw7	LD107
HLA-Dw8	LD108
HLA-Dw9	TB9, OH
HLA-Dw10	LD16
HLA-Dw11	LD17

Table 4. Nomenclature for the new specificities established by serological assays on B lymphocytes

New nomenclature	7th Workshop nomenclature [a]
DRw1	WIA1
DRw2	WIA2
DRw3	WIA3
DRw4	WIA4
DRw5	WIA5
DRw6	WIA6
DRw7	WIA7

[a] Other equivalent nomenclatures and further details concerning the definition of these specificities can be found in Bodmer et al. (*4*).

(previously LD17) appears to be more or less included in HLA-Dw7 and may turn out to be a " split " of this latter specificity.

Other suggested specificities discussed but not yet considered ready for provisional w designation, pending further cell exchanges evaluated by appropriate statistical procedures, were RE and the Japanese specificities HO and YT or AW. Further exchanges are also needed before other suggested MLC loci, possibly distinct from HLA-D, can be considered. At the 6th and 7th Workshops on Histocompatibility Testing a group of reference laboratories for cellular typing was established, on an informal basis, and these laboratories are continuing to collaborate in cell exchanges in order to clarify the definition of these and other proposed specifities (*4*).

Specificities identified by serological techniques on B lymphocytes

The 7th Workshop consolidated a major advance in the definition of the new specificities identified by serological techniques on B lymphocytes, mainly using a microlymphocytotoxicity assay on purified peripheral blood B lymphocytes. These specificities, which appear to be the counterpart of at least some of the so called Ia determinants of the mouse major histocompatibility system, H-2, are in general closely associated with the already defined specificities of the HLA-D locus. In order to reflect this relationship, while at the same time reserving judgement on whether these serologically detected determinants are on the products of the HLA-D locus, it has been decided to use for them the designation DR (for D related), followed, as usual, by the letter w to indicate that the designation is still provisional. This nomenclature for the first seven DRw specificities, using numbers that correspond to the relevant associated Dw specificity, is given in Table 4, together with their 7th Workshop equivalents. The specificities DRw1, DRw2, DRw3, and DRw7 are clearly defined, each by several sera. DRw4 has been defined in two ways. First, by sera that show some evidence of cross-reaction with DRw5 but do not consistently react with any other specificity; second, by sera that contain activity against DRw4 and DRw7, and so can be used to define DRw4 only in the absence of DRw7, again reflecting cross-reaction, in this case between DRw4 and DRw7. The specificity DRw6 is the least well defined, as the available sera react in addition either with DRw3 and possibly DRw5, or with DRw2 and often also DRw1. These cross-reaction patterns, which seem to be a common feature of the DRw specificities, may reflect the existence of supertypic specificities for, for example, the combinations DRw1, DRw2, and DRw6, or DRw4, DRw5, and possibly DRw7. Allowing for these problems of cross-reaction, the evidence so far is consistent with the hypothesis that these seven specificities are controlled genetically by a single multiple allelic series, as in the case of the HLA-A, B, C, and D loci.

In the 7th Workshop, an effort was made to define an HLA-Dw8 associated specificity (Workshop designation WIA8) but this was considered to be not yet sufficiently well established to be assigned a provisional w designation. There were, in addition, a number of suggestions for other specificities, mainly identified as " tails " in the 7th Workshop sera, and these also need further evaluation before they can be considered for a w designation. Some evidence has been obtained, both before and during the Workshop, for the existence of one or more determinants coded for by a locus in the neighbourhood of HLA-A, but once again further work is needed before this can be considered for a new locus symbol. It is probable that, in due course, serological tests on B

Table 5. Complete listing of recognized HLA specificities [a]

HLA-A	HLA-B		HLA-C	HLA-D	HLA-DR
HLA-A1	HLA-B5	HLA-Bw42	HLA-Cw1	HLA-Dw1	HLA-DRw1
HLA-A2	HLA-B7	HLA-Bw44	HLA-Cw2	HLA-Dw2	HLA-DRw2
HLA-A3	HLA-B8	HLA-Bw45	HLA-Cw3	HLA-Dw3	HLA-DRw3
HLA-A9	HLA-B12	HLA-Bw46	HLA-Cw4	HLA-Dw4	HLA-DRw4
HLA-A10	HLA-B13	HLA-Bw47	HLA-Cw5	HLA-Dw5	HLA-DRw5
HLA-A11	HLA-B14	HLA-Bw48	HLA-Cw6	HLA-Dw6	HLA-DRw6
HLA-Aw19	HLA-B15	HLA-Bw49		HLA-Dw7	HLA-DRw7
HLA-Aw23	HLA-Bw16	HLA-Bw50		HLA-Dw8	
HLA-Aw24	HLA-B17	HLA-Bw51		HLA-Dw9	
HLA-A25	HLA-B18	HLA-Bw52		HLA-Dw10	
HLA-A26	HLA-Bw21	HLA-Bw53		HLA-Dw11	
HLA-A28	HLA-Bw22	HLA-Bw54			
HLA-A29	HLA-B27				
HLA-Aw30	HLA-Bw35				
HLA-Aw31	HLA-B37				
HLA-Aw32	HLA-Bw38				
HLA-Aw33	HLA-Bw39				
HLA-Aw34	HLA-B40				
HLA-Aw36	HLA-Bw41				
HLA-Aw43					
	HLA-Bw4				
	HLA-Bw6				

[a] The following specificities arose as clear-cut splits of other specifities:

HLA-A9	into	HLA-Aw23	HLA-Aw24
HLA-A10	into	HLA-A25	HLA-A26
HLA-B5	into	HLA-Bw51	HLA-Bw52
HLA-B12	into	HLA-Bw44	HLA-Bw45
HLA-Bw16	into	HLA-Bw38	HLA-Bw39
HLA-Bw21	into	HLA-Bw49	HLA-Bw5

Historically HLA-Aw19 has included HLA-A29, HLA-Aw30, HLA-Aw31, HLA-Aw32, and HLA-Aw33.

lymphocytes and other techniques including, for example, the primed lymphocyte test (PLT) and cell-mediated lymphocytotoxicity (CML) may define other loci in and outside the HLA region. Though evidence has been obtained that suggests a relatively close relation between determinants identified using the PLT test and the DRw and similar specificities, the results of the 7th Workshop exchange did not warrant the designation of any separate nomenclature for these.

The committee adheres to the view that it should confine its attention to the cell surface determinants, identified by serological and cellular techniques, that are coded for by genes in the HLA region. This does not exclude the possibility that it may in the future have to broaden its horizon beyond the HLA region. However, the committee reaffirms its recommendation that the pre-emption of formal symbols, such as HLB, HL-B or HLA-E, that are clearly related to the symbols used in the nomenclature for factors of the HLA system, is to be strongly discouraged before their use has been considered by the committee.

The members of the committee accept that their laboratories should play a major role in the exchanges of sera, cells, and information that are needed to continue to clarify the definition of new and proposed factors of the HLA system. This cooperation provides a network of reference laboratories that can, together with the workshops, continue to aid the clear development of knowledge of the HLA system.

* * *

E. Albert, University Polyclinic for Children, Munich, Federal Republic of Germany.

D. B. Amos, Duke Medical Center, Durham, NC, USA (*Chairman*)

W. F. Bodmer, Genetics Laboratory, University of Oxford, Oxford, England (*Rapporteur*)

R. Ceppellini, Institute for Immunology, Basle, Switzerland, and CNR Centre for the Study of Immunogenetics and Histocompatibility, Turin, Italy

J. Dausset, Institut de Recherches sur les Maladies du Sang, Hôpital Saint-Louis, Paris, France.

F. Kissmeyer-Nielsen, The University Hospital, Aarhus, Denmark.

W. Mayr, Institut for Blood Group Serology, University of Vienna, Vienna, Austria.
R. Payne, Stanford University School of Medicine, Stanford, CA, USA.
J. J. van Rood, University of Leiden, Netherlands.
P. I. Terasaki, University of California School of Medicine, Los Angeles, CA, USA.
Z. Trnka, Institute for Immunology, Basle, Switzerland, representing Immunology, Division of Noncommunicable Diseases, World Health Organization, and the IUIS Nomenclature Committee (*Secretary*).
R. L. Walford, University of California School of Medicine, Los Angeles, CA, USA.

ACKNOWLEDGEMENTS

The contributions of Julia Bodmer and Hilliard Festenstein, who acted as co-opted members of the committee for the meeting that led to the preparation of this report, are gratefully acknowledged.

REFERENCES

1. *Bulletin of the World Health Organization*, **39**: 483 (1968).
2. *Bulletin of the World Health Organization*, **47**: 659 (1972).
3. *Bulletin of the World Health Organization*, **52**: 261 (1975).
4. Bodmer, W. F. et al., ed. *Histocompatibility testing*. Copenhagen, Munksgaard, 1977.

Nomenclature for factors of the HLA system, 1980*

This article outlines the decisions made by the WHO nomenclature committee on leukocyte antigens at a meeting held after the 8th International Workshop on Histocompatibility Testing. Particular attention is given to new designations for provisional HLA-B and HLA-DR specificities and the upgrading of certain HLA-D and HLA-DR specificities to full HLA status. The existence of supertypic cross-reacting specificities was confirmed and extended.

The HLA nomenclature committee met under the auspices of the World Health Organization and the International Union of Immunological Societies, after the 8th International Histocompatibility Testing Workshop, in order to consider revisions and additions to the nomenclature following the principles established in previous reports (*1–5*).

HLA-A, HLA-B, and HLA-C specificities

There are no changes or additions to the nomenclature for the HLA-A specificities.

There are no changes to the nomenclature for the previously identified HLA-B specificities. New designations for provisional HLA-B specificities are listed in Table 1. All are subdivisions or "splits" of previously identified specificities. At present, Bw59 (defined by extra reactions of some B8 antisera) is found predominantly in Oriental populations. The following suggested specificities were considered, but the committee felt that they were not sufficiently well defined to be given a provisional designation: 8w57[a] (Bf, SN-2, Te90), 8w58 (5y, Te73), 8w59 (Bu, SV, K5, DA(6), 8w62 (14.2), 8w63 (14.1), 8w66 (Te74, 15.3).

As there has been no change in the nomenclature for the complement components coded for by genes in the HLA region, it has been decided to retain the Cw nomenclature for all the HLA-C locus specificities (*4*), even though Cw1, Cw2, Cw3, Cw4, and Cw5 are sufficiently well defined to justify upgrading to full HLA nomenclature status. Cw6 remains difficult to define, especially in the presence of Cw4. Two new HLA-Cw specificities are given in Table 2.

Table 1. New designations for provisional specificities of the HLA-B locus

New	Previous equivalents	8th Workshop nomenclature
HLA-Bw55	22.1	8w55
HLA-Bw56	22.2, Te92, Da30	8w56
HLA-Bw57	17.1, 17A, 17 long	8w67
HLA-Bw58	17.2, 17B, 17 short	8w68
HLA-Bw59	HOK-1, 8.2'	8w69
HLA-Bw60	40.1	8w60
HLA-Bw61	40.2	8w61
HLA-Bw62	15.1, To53, 15B, Te72	8w64
HLA-Bw63	15.2, To52, 15A, Te71	8w65

Table 2. New designations for provisional specificities of the HLA-C locus

New	Previous equivalents	8th Workshop nomenclature
HLA-Cw7	Cve, CTo-1	8wCw7
HLA-Cw8	T8, T9	8wCw8, 8wCw9

* The report of the HLA nomenclature committee was first published in *Tissue antigens*, **16**: 113-117 (1980). This terminology note, which was drafted by the signatories listed on page 946, is based on the report and is published by permission of Munksgaard International Publishers Ltd., Copenhagen. A French translation will be published in a future issue of the *Bulletin*.

[a] 8w57, etc., were designations used during the 8th Workshop (*6*).

HLA-D specificities

The definition of the specificities Dw1, Dw2, Dw3, and Dw5 has improved but is still not good enough to allow the provisional w designation to be dropped. The inclusion of Dw11 in Dw7 was confirmed during the 8th Workshop, although Dw7 itself is difficult to define. The identification of Dw10 was much improved, whereas Dw4, Dw6, Dw8, and Dw9 are still poorly defined, with clear indications of heterogeneity for Dw4 and Dw6. One new specificity was defined in Oriental populations, namely HLA-Dw12, formerly DH0 or DB4 (8th Workshop designations) (*6*).

Other specificities discussed, but considered not sufficiently well defined to be given a provisional designation, include DB1 (associated with Dw7), DB2 (associated with Dw5), DB3, and DB5 (8th Workshop designations) (*6*).

HLA-DR specificities

The DR specificities upgraded to full HLA status are listed in Table 3. DRw6 retains its provisional status since the lack of operationally monospecific antisera makes its definition difficult. Three new provisional specificities are listed in Table 4. While the correlation between the previously well-established D and DR specificities remains unambiguous, it has become clear that the definition of new specificities has made it difficult to maintain the parallelism between the D and DR nomenclature. Thus DRw9 and DRw10 are not specifically associated with Dw9 and Dw10. Other specificities discussed, but not considered sufficiently well defined to be given a provisional designation, included 8w13, YYY or 5/6, and various suggested subdivisions of DRw6.

The existence of supertypic cross-reacting specificities, which had been partially identified during the 7th workshop (*5*), was confirmed during the 8th Workshop. The combinations (DR1, DR2, DRw6, DRw10), (DR3, DR5, DRw6, DRw8), and (DR4, DR7, DRw9) were noted and given the designations MT1 (DC1), MT2, and MT3, respectively (*6*). It is not yet clear whether these supertypic antigens and certain other specificities discussed in the report of the 8th Workshop (*6*) are on the currently recognized DR locus molecular products, or on other locus products, or both. These, and other problems of definition of combinations of specificities need to be clarified by further analysis of the serological and genetic data and by other approaches, such as the use of monoclonal antibodies and detailed biochemical analysis.

Table 3. New designations for HLA-DR specificities that have been upgraded to full HLA status

New	Previous
HLA-DR1	HLA-DRw1
HLA-DR2	HLA-DRw2
HLA-DR3	HLA-DRw3
HLA-DR4	HLA-DRw4
HLA-DR5	HLA-DRw5
HLA-DR7	HLA-DRw7

Table 4. New designations for provisional specificities of the HLA-DR locus

New	Previous equivalents	8th Workshop nomenclature
HLA-DRw8	WIA8	8wDRw8
HLA-DRw9	WIA4x7, DuB15	8wDRw12 included DRw9 and DRw10
HLA-DRw10	ST-1, LTM	8wDRw14

* * *

E. Albert, Kinderpoliklinik der Universität, Munich, Germany
D. B. Amos, Duke Medical Center, Durham, NC, USA (*Chairman*)
W. F. Bodmer, Imperial Cancer Research Fund Laboratories, London, England (*Rapporteur*)
R. Ceppellini, Institute for Immunology, Basel, Switzerland
J. Dausset, Institut de Recherches sur les Maladies du Sang, Hôpital Saint-Louis, Paris, France
F. Kissmeyer-Nielsen, The University Hospital, Aarhus, Denmark
W. Mayr, Institut für Blutgruppenserologie, Vienna University, Vienna, Austria
R. Payne, Stanford University School of Medicine, Stanford, California, USA (*Rapporteur*)
J. J. van Rood, University of Leiden, Leiden, The Netherlands
P. I. Terasaki, UCLA School of Medicine, University of California, Los Angeles, California, USA
R. L. Walford, UCLA School of Medicine, University of California, Los Angeles, California, USA

Table 5. Complete listing of recognized HLA specificities[a]

HLA-A	HLA-B	HLA-C	HLA-D	HLA-DR
HLA-A1	HLA-B5	HLA-Cw1	HLA-Dw1	HLA-DR1
HLA-A2	HLA-B7	HLA-Cw2	HLA-Dw2	HLA-DR2
HLA-A3	HLA-B8	HLA-Cw3	HLA-Dw3	HLA-DR3
HLA-A9	HLA-B12	HLA-Cw4	HLA-Dw4	HLA-DR4
HLA-A10	HLA-B13	HLA-Cw5	HLA-Dw5	HLA-DR5
HLA-A11	HLA-B14	HLA-Cw6	HLA-Dw6	HLA-DRw6
HLA-Aw19	HLA-B15	HLA-Cw7	HLA-Dw7	HLA-DR7
HLA-Aw23(9)	HLA-Bw16	HLA-Cw8	HLA-Dw8	HLA-DRw8
HLA-Aw24(9)	HLA-B17		HLA-Dw9	HLA-DRw9
HLA-A25(10)	HLA-B18		HLA-Dw10	HLA-DRw10
HLA-A26(10)	HLA-Bw21		HLA-Dw11	
HLA-A28	HLA-Bw22		HLA-Dw12	
HLA-A29	HLA-B27			
HLA-Aw30	HLA-Bw35			
HLA-Aw31	HLA-B37			
HLA-Aw32	HLA-Bw38(w16)			
HLA-Aw33	HLA-Bw39(w16)			
HLA-Aw34	HLA-B40			
HLA-Aw36	HLA-Bw41			
HLA-Aw43	HLA-Bw42			
	HLA-Bw44(12)			
	HLA-Bw45(12)			
	HLA-Bw46			
	HLA-Bw47			
	HLA-Bw48			
	HLA-Bw49(w21)			
	HLA-Bw50(w21)			
	HLA-Bw51(5)			
	HLA-Bw52(5)			
	HLA-Bw53			
	HLA-Bw54(w22)			
	HLA-Bw55(w22)			
	HLA-Bw56(w22)			
	HLA-Bw57(17)			
	HLA-Bw58(17)			
	HLA-Bw59			
	HLA-Bw60(40)			
	HLA-Bw61(40)			
	HLA-Bw62(15)			
	HLA-Bw63(15)			
	HLA-Bw4[b]			
	HLA-Bw6			

[a] The listing of broad specificities in parentheses after a narrow specificity, e.g., HLA-Aw23(9) is optional. The following arose as clear-cut splits of other specificities.

HLA-A9	into	Aw23, Aw24
HLA-A10	into	A25, A26
HLA-B5	into	Bw51, Bw52
HLA-B12	into	Bw44, Bw45
HLA-B15	into	Bw62, Bw63
HLA-Bw16	into	Bw38, Bw39
HLA-B17	into	Bw57, Bw58
HLA-Bw21	into	Bw49, Bw50
HLA-Bw22	into	Bw54, Bw55, Bw56
HLA-B40	into	Bw60, Bw61

[b] The following are the generally agreed inclusions of HLA-B specificities in Bw4 and Bw6:

Bw4: B13, B27, B37, Bw38(w16), Bw44(12), Bw47, Bw49(w21), Bw51(5), Bw52(5), Bw53, Bw57(17), Bw58(17), Bw59, Bw63(15)

Bw6: B7, B8, B14, B18, Bw35, Bw39(16), Bw41, Bw42, Bw45(12), Bw46, Bw48, Bw50(w21), Bw54(w22), Bw55(w22), Bw56(w22), Bw60(40), Bw61(40), Bw62(15).

ACKNOWLEDGEMENTS

The contributions of Dr Domenico Bernoco, Dr Min Sik Park, Dr M. R. Mickey, Dr Bo Dupont, and Dr Edmund Yunis, who acted as co-opted members of the committee for the meeting that led to the preparation of this report, are gratefully acknowledged.

REFERENCES

1. *Bulletin of the World Health Organization*, **39**: 483 (1968).
2. *Bulletin of the World Health Organization*, **47**: 659 (1972).
3. *Bulletin of the World Health Organization*, **52**: 261 (1975).
4. *Bulletin of the World Health Organization*, **56**: 461 (1978).
5. BODMER, W. ET AL., ed., *Histocompatibility testing 1977*. Copenhagen, Munksgaard, 1978.
6. TERASAKI, P. I., ed., *Histocompatibility testing 1980*. Los Angeles, California, UCLA Tissue Typing Laboratory, 1980.

Nomenclature for factors of the HLA system, 1984*

This article presents the decisions of the nomenclature committee on leukocyte antigens, which met in Vienna on 16–17 May 1984.

The HLA nomenclature committee met under the auspices of the World Health Organization, after the Ninth International Histocompatibility Testing Workshop which was held in Munich and Vienna on 6–15 May 1984, to consider revisions and additions to the nomenclature of factors identified by serological and cellular typing following the principles established successively in previous reports (*1-6*). The nomenclature for the variants of the complement components controlled by genes of the HLA region was not considered, as it was assumed that this was the responsibility of those with a special interest in complement (see reference 7). Special attention was given to establishing a revised system of nomenclature for the products (sometimes called class II) of what can now be called the HLA-D region, based on the recent advances in our understanding of the biochemistry and genetics of these products.

The decision to upgrade a specificity, namely to drop its "w" designation, took into account the correlation in the overall workshop data between the local laboratory assignment of a specificity and that arrived at by the central computer analysis. A correlation coefficient of around 0.95 or higher, together with general availability of appropriate antisera, was taken as a sufficient indication of adequate clarity of definition of a specificity to drop the "w" designation. This criterion was applied equally to broader and narrower specificities even though, in some cases, the splits of the broader specificity were not so well defined. This is, for example, still the case for HLA-B5 with its splits B51 and Bw52. The retention of a "w" in the designation remains an indication that the specificity, though clearly identified, may not always be easily defined.

HLA-A, HLA-B, and HLA-C specificities

As before, the HLA-A and HLA-B specificities are numbered jointly with non-overlapping numbers. The "w" designation is retained for all HLA-C specificities to avoid confusion with the nomenclature for complement components.

Newly upgraded HLA-A and HLA-B specificities are listed in Table 1. In addition to Cw1, Cw2, Cw3, Cw4 and Cw5, Cw6 approaches the clarity of definition that would be required for dropping the "w" designation. However, Cw5 remains slightly more difficult to define than Cw1, Cw2, Cw3 or Cw4.

New provisional designations for HLA-A and HLA-B specificities are listed in Tables 2 and 3 respectively. Aw66 (previously LN) is effectively another split of A10 and cannot so far be defined serologically in the presence of A26. Aw69 (previously A2/28) is a split of A28 that is most clearly defined by monoclonal antibodies with reactivity only against A2 and Aw69, and cannot so far be defined serologically in the presence of A2. This is the first example of an officially recognized specificity identified by a monoclonal antibody. Given the potential exquisite specificity of monoclonal antibodies, criteria for the designation of new specificities identified by them need careful consideration. Aw69 has been designated because at least two monoclonal antibodies agree in defining a new specificity that is clearly distinct from any previously identified specificity. Aw68 is defined as the split of A28 that is complementary to Aw69. Since Bw71 (previously Bu) and Bw72 (previously SV) cannot always be distinguished serologically from each other, it was also necessary to designate the broad specificity Bw70 (previously

* A French translation of this article appears on pages 407-413. The names of the members of the committee that prepared this note are given on pages 402 and 405. Requests for reprints should be sent to Chief, Immunology, World Health Organization, 1211 Geneva 27, Switzerland.

Table 1. New designations for HLA-A and HLA-B specificities that have been upgraded to full HLA status

New	Previous equivalents
A23	Aw23
A24	Aw24
A30	Aw30
A31	Aw31
A32	Aw32
B16	Bw16
B21	Bw21
B35	Bw35
B38	Bw38
B39	Bw39
B44	Bw44
B45	Bw45
B49	Bw49
B51	Bw51

Table 2. New provisional designations of HLA-A specificities

New	Previous equivalents
Aw66	LN
Aw68	A28 and negative to A2/28
Aw69	A2/28

Table 3. New provisional designations for HLA-B specificities

New	Previous equivalents
Bw64	B14.1, (8w63)
Bw65	B14.2, (8w62)
Bw67	SN-2, Te90, (8w57), Te75
Bw70	Bu + SV, K5, Da(6), (8w59)
Bw71	Bu
Bw72	SV
Bw73	KA, IEH

Bu + SV, K5 or Da(6)).

Other suggested HLA-A or HLA-B specificities discussed, but not yet considered to be sufficiently well defined to merit official provisional designation, included 9.3, Th (a possible further split of Aw19 in negroid populations), 19bac, 33.1, 33.2, St16 (a possible further split of B39), 15.3 and Te74 (another B15 split sometimes referred to as 8w66, an informal designation that should be avoided to prevent any possible confusion with Aw66). Special attention clearly needs to be given to clarification of the many possible further splits of B15, seen especially in oriental populations.

Individual workshop sera suggested a new specificity that may fill part of the HLA-C blank, and a split of Cw3. Other sera suggested splits of Cw7. However, none of these suggestions were considered to be sufficiently well founded to merit an official provisional designation. The combination of Cw1 and Cw3, seen in association with haplotypes containing Bw46, was not given a separate designation as it is not yet clear whether this is simply a reflection of gene duplication (in whole or in part) or truly represents a novel serological specificity.

The HLA-D region

Biochemical and molecular genetical analyses of the products and genes associated with the HLA-Dw and HLA-DR(w) specificities have led to a considerable advance in our understanding of the HLA-D region and its products. It is now clear that there are at least three well-defined subsets of products, which until now have been informally designated as DR, DC (MB or DS) and SB. Each product consists of a non-covalently associated combination of an α- and a β-chain. The α and β chains are substantially different from each other, and there is evidence for at least six α chain genes and seven β chain genes all in the HLA region. These genes, for the most part, appear to be arranged in subsets corresponding to the three subsets of products, where α and β chain genes within a subset are significantly more similar to each other than they are to the genes of one of the other subsets. While present knowledge concerning the genes of the HLA-D region is not yet adequate to give them each an official designation, it was decided that the division into three subsets of products is sufficiently well established to merit an official designation and that this could be done without prejudicing future decisions on nomenclature for the specificities and genes of the HLA-D region. The chosen designations are HLA-DR, HLA-DQ (previously DC, etc.), and HLA-DP (previously SB). Current evidence suggests one α and two or three β chain genes for HLA-DR, and two α and two β chains each for HLA-DQ and HLA-DP. It is anticipated that when eventually gene names are officially designated they will consist of HLA-DR, HLA-DQ, HLA-DP, followed by a combination of numbers and letters (A for an α-chain gene and B for a β-chain gene) that uniquely defines each gene. The HLA-D region is the counterpart of the I-region of the mouse H-2 system, whose determinants are sometimes called Ia, with I-A corresponding to DQ, and I-E to DR.

The serologically defined specificities of the HLA-D region can be associated predominantly with either the HLA-DR or HLA-DQ sets of products, while the different HLA-DP products are so far only defined using the primed lymphocyte test (or PLT). Certain monomorphic monoclonal antibodies can, however, clearly distinguish between these three sets of products.

The HLA-Dw specificities, defined by the mixed lymphocyte culture (or MLC) test, cannot yet be clearly associated with one or other of the three subsets of products, though it seems likely that they mostly involve HLA-DR. Where new specificities are clearly identified as being associated predominantly with one or other of the subsets of HLA-D products, we have followed previous practice in assigning to them the designation HLA-DR, HLA-DQ or HLA-DP (followed by "w" to indicate that the designation is provisional) and appropriate numbers, usually in sequence. The designation HLA-Dw, with no further indication of subdivisions, is retained for the MLC-defined specificities.

Table 4. New provisional designations for HLA-DR specificities

New	Previous equivalents
DRw11	LB5
DRw12	LB5x8, DR5 short, FT23
DRw13	6.6, 6.1, 6Z
DRw14	6.9, 6.3, 6X, 901
DRw52	MT2
DRw53	MT3

Table 5. New provisional designations of HLA-DQ specificities

New	Previous equivalents
DQw1	DC1, MB1, MT1, LB-E12
DQw2	MB2, DC3, Te24, LB-E17
DQw3	MB3, MT4, DC4, TB21

HLA-DR specificities

The previously defined HLA-DR1, DR2, DR3, DR4, DR5, DRw6, DR7, DRw8, DRw9, and DRw10 specificities are all clearly associated with the HLA-DR products. They therefore retain their previous designations, since it was decided that none of DRw6, DRw8, DRw9 or DRw10 deserved to be upgraded to full HLA status. Amongst HLA-DR specificities with full HLA status, DR5 remains the most difficult to define.

New provisional designations for HLA-DR specificities are given in Table 4. DRw11 (previously LB5) and DRw12 (previously LB5x8, etc.) are splits of DR5, while DRw13 (previously 6.6, 6.1, 6Z) and DRw14 (previously 6.3, 6.9, 6X, 901) are splits of DRw6.

DRw52 (previously MT2) and DRw53 (previously MT3) were originally identified in the 7th and 8th Workshops as apparently cross-reacting specificities involving DR3, DR5, DRw6 and DRw8 for DRw52, and DR4, DR7 and DRw9 for DRw53. Following the 8th Workshop, it was suggested that these two specificities might be on molecules from a different locus (sometimes also referred to as BR) to that controlling the then designated HLA-DR specificities, or possibly on molecules from both the then assumed HLA-DR locus and another locus, and this remains true. But it is now clear that all such molecules must be members of the HLA-DR subset. High numbers were chosen for these two broad, operationally supertypic, specificities to separate them clearly from the other, narrower HLA-DR specificities. DRw6, in particular, seems operationally to be completely included in DRw52 (previously MT2).

Other suggested HLA-DR specificities that were discussed, but not yet considered to be sufficiently well defined to merit official provisional designation, included 4.1, 4.2, 4.3, and DR2 splits.

HLA-DQ specificities

New provisional HLA-DQ specificities are listed in Table 5. As in the case of DRw52 (previously MT2) and DRw53 (previously MT3), DQw1 (previously DC1, MB1, MT1, LB-E12), DQw2 (previously MB2, DC3, Te24, LB-E17), and DQw3 (previously MB3, MT4, DC4, TB21) were originally identified in the 7th and 8th Workshops as apparently cross-reacting specificities including DR1, DR2, DRw6 and DRw10 for DQw1, DR3 and DR7 for DQw2, and DR4 and DR5 for DQw3. These were also suggested at the time of the 8th Workshop to be on different locus products from the HLA-DR specificities. Subsequent studies, in this case, have clearly associated these specificities with the HLA-DQ (previously DC, etc.) products. TA10 and LB-E13 were discussed as possible HLA-DQ specificities, apparently splitting DQw3, but it was felt that their relationship with HLA-DQ products required some further independent confirmation, and so they were not assigned official provisional designations.

The fact that DQw1 (previously DC1, etc.) and DRw6 are on different sets of products clearly

Table 6. New provisional designations for HLA-DP specificities

New	Previous equivalents
DPw1	SB1, PL3A
DPw2	SB2
DPw3	SB3
DPw4	SB4, PL3B
DPw5	SB5
DPw6	SB6

indicates that DQw1 does not contribute to the definition of DRw6. The strong population associations between these and other analogous combinations of specificities can now be seen clearly to be due to strong linkage disequilibrium between alleles at very closely linked loci coding for DR and DQ products.

HLA-DP specificities

New provisional HLA-DP specificities, as defined by PLT typing, are listed in Table 6.

Table 7. New provisional designations for HLA-Dw specificities

New	Previous equivalents
Dw13	DB3
Dw14	LD40
Dw15	DYT, YT
Dw16	DB8, B8
Dw17	7A, (Dw7A)
Dw18	6A, (Dw6A)
Dw19	6B, (Dw6B)

Table 8. Dw and DR relationships

Dw specificities	Associated DR specificities
Dw1	DR1
Dw2, Dw12	DR2
Dw3	DR3
Dw4, Dw10, Dw13, Dw14, Dw15	DR4
Dw5	DRw11 (5)
Dw6, Dw18, Dw19	DRw13 (w6)
Dw9, Dw16	DRw14 (w6)
Dw7, Dw11, Dw17	DR7
Dw8	DRw8

HLA-Dw specificities

HLA-Dw1, Dw2 and Dw3 now approach the clarity of definition by MLC typing that would justify dropping their "w" designation. However, in order to distinguish the MLC-identified specificities from those clearly assigned to one of the HLA-D region products it was decided, at least for the time being, to use the prefix Dw for all the MLC-identified specificities, however well defined they are.

New provisional designations for HLA-Dw specificities are listed in Table 7. Dw13 (previously DB3), Dw14 (previously LD40), and Dw15 (previously DYT, found predominantly in oriental populations), together with Dw4 and Dw10, are all associated with the serological specificity DR4. Dw2 and Dw12 have similarly previously been associated with DR2. Dw17 (previously 7A) is the complementary split of Dw7 to Dw11, while Dw18 (previously 6A) and Dw19 (previously 6B) are splits of Dw6, which is in turn associated with the serological specificity DRw13, one of the splits of DRw6. The other split of DRw6, DRw14, is associated with Dw9 and Dw16. These multiple relationships between Dw and DR specificities, further confounded by patterns of association with DQ specificities that are probably due to linkage disequilibrium between alleles at DR and DQ loci, emphasize again that it is no longer possible to maintain any relationship between the numbering of Dw and DR specificities. A list of the known relationships between officially designated Dw and DR specificities is given in Table 8.

Other specificities not officially designated included DB6 (originally defined by the cell Herluf), DB9, and a split of Dw8, informally called 8.2, which appears to occur especially in Eskimo and American-Indian populations. These specificities, probably for technical reasons, were not well defined in the final workshop analysis.

A complete listing of the recognized HLA specificities is given in Table 9. Further background to the basis for the decisions reported here can be found in *Histocompatibility testing 1984* (*8*).

*

* *

W. F. Bodmer, Imperial Cancer Research Fund, London, England (*Rapporteur*).

E. Albert, Polyclinic for Children, University of Munich, Federal Republic of Germany.

J. G. Bodmer, Imperial Cancer Research Fund, London, England.

J. Dausset, Institut de Recherches sur les Maladies du Sang, Hôpital Saint Louis, Paris, France.

F. Kissmeyer-Nielsen, The University Hospital, Aarhus, Denmark.

Table 9. Complete listing of recognized HLA specificities

HLA-A	HLA-B	HLA-C	HLA-D	HLA-DR	HLA-DQ	HLA-DP
A1	B5	Cw1	Dw1	DR1	DQw1	DPw1
A2	B7	Cw2	Dw2	DR2	DQw2	DPw2
A3	B8	Cw3	Dw3	DR3	DQw3	DPw3
A9	B12	Cw4	Dw4	DR4		DPw4
A10	B13	Cw5	Dw5	DR5		DPw5
A11	B14	Cw6	Dw6	DRw6		DPw6
Aw19	B15	Cw7	Dw7	DR7		
A23(9) [a]	B16	Cw8	Dw8	DRw8		
A24(9)	B17		Dw9	DRw9		
A25(10)	B18		Dw10	DRw10		
A26(10)	B21		Dw11(w7) [a]	DRw11(5) [a]		
A28	Bw22		Dw12	DRw12(5)		
A29(w19)	B27		Dw13	DRw13(w6)		
A30(w19)	B35		Dw14	DRw14(w6)		
A31(w19)	B37		Dw15			
A32(w19)	B38(16) [a]		Dw16	DRw52 [c]		
Aw33(w19)	B39(16)		Dw17(w7)	DRw53 [c]		
Aw34(10)	B40		Dw18(w6)			
Aw36	Bw41		Dw19(w6)			
Aw43	Bw42					
Aw66(10)	B44(12)					
Aw68(28)	B45(12)					
Aw69(28)	Bw46					
	Bw47					
	Bw48					
	Bw49(21)					
	Bw50(21)					
	B51(5)					
	Bw52(5)					
	Bw53					
	Bw54(w22)					
	Bw55(w22)					
	Bw56(w22)					
	Bw57(17)					
	Bw58(17)					
	Bw59					
	Bw60(40)					
	Bw61(40)					
	Bw62(15)					
	Bw63(15)					
	Bw64(14)					
	Bw65(14)					
	Bw67					
	Bw70					
	Bw71(w70)					
	Bw72(w70)					
	Bw73					
	Bw4 [b]					
	Bw6 [b]					

(Table 9: *continued on next page*)

Table 9: *continued*

[a] The listing of broad specificities in parentheses after a narrow specificity, e.g., HLA-A23(9), is optional. The following is a listing of those specificities which arose as clear-cut splits of other specificities:

Original broad specificities	*Splits*
A9	A23, A24
A10	A25, A26, Aw34, Aw66
Aw19	A29, A30, A31, A32, Aw33
A28	Aw68, Aw69
B5	B51, Bw52
B12	B44, B45
B14	Bw64, Bw65
B15	Bw62, Bw63
B16	B38, B39
B17	Bw57, Bw58
B21	B49, Bw50
Bw22	Bw54, Bw55, Bw56
B40	Bw60, Bw61
Bw70	Bw71, Bw72
DR5	DRw11, DRw12
DRw6	DRw13, DRw14
Dw6	Dw18, Dw19
Dw7	Dw11, Dw17

[b] The following are the generally agreed inclusions of HLA-B specificities into Bw4 and Bw6:

Bw4: B5, B13, B17, B27, B37, B38(16), B44(12), Bw47, B49(21), B51(5), Bw52(5), Bw53, Bw57(17), Bw58(17), Bw59, Bw63(15).
Bw6: B7, B8, B14, B18, Bw22, B35, B39(16), B40, Bw41, Bw42, B45(12), Bw46, Bw48, Bw50(21), Bw54(w22), Bw55(w22), Bw56(w22), Bw60(40), Bw61(40), Bw62(15), Bw64(14), Bw65(14), Bw67, Bw70, Bw71(w70), Bw72(w70), Bw73.

[c] The following specificities are generally agreed to be associated with DRw52 and DRw53:

DRw52: DR3, DR5, DRw6, DRw8, DRw11(5), DRw12(5), DRw13(w6), DRw14(w6)
DRw53: DR4, DR7, DRw9.

W. Mayr, Institute for Blood Group Serology, University of Vienna, Vienna, Austria.
R. Payne, Stanford University School of Medicine, Stanford, CA, USA.
J. J. van Rood, University of Leiden, Leiden, Netherlands (*Chairman*).
Z. Trnka, Institute for Immunology, Basle, Switzerland.
R. L. Walford, University of California School of Medicine, Los Angeles, CA, USA.

ACKNOWLEDGEMENTS

The contributions of Dr Max Baur, Dr Hans-Grosse Wilde, and Dr Ieke Schreuder, who acted as co-opted members of the committee that produced this report, are gratefully acknowledged.

REFERENCES

1. *Bulletin of the World Health Organization*, **39**: 483 (1968).
2. TERASAKI, P. I., ed., *Histocompatibility testing 1970*, Copenhagen, Munksgaard, 1970, p. 49.
3. *Bulletin of the World Health Organization*, **47**: 659 (1972).
4. *Bulletin of the World Health Organization*, **52**: 261 (1975).
5. *Bulletin of the World Health Organization*, **56**: 461 (1978).
6. TERASAKI, P. I. ed., *Histocompatibility testing 1980*, Los Angeles, UCLA Tissue Typing Laboratory, 1980, pp. 18-20.
7. MAUFF, G. ET AL., Statement on the nomenclature of human C4 allotypes. *Immunobiology*, **164**: 184-191 (1983).
8. ALBERT, E. D. ET AL., ed., *Histocompatibility testing 1984*, Heidelberg, Springer Verlag, 1984.

HLA Antigens

Nomenclature for Factors of the HLA System, 1996

Julia G. Bodmer, Steven G. E. Marsh, Ekkehard D. Albert, Walter F. Bodmer, Ronald E. Bontrop, Dominique Charron, Bo Dupont, Henry A. Erlich, Renee Fauchet, Bernard Mach, Wolfgang R. Mayr, Peter Parham, Takehiko Sasazuki, Geziena M. Th. Schreuder, Jack L. Strominger, Arne Svejgaard and Paul I. Terasaki*/**

The WHO Nomenclature Committee for Factors of the HLA System met in the Institut Biomédical des Cordeliers, in Paris in June 1996 after the 12th International Histocompatibility Workshop and Conference to consider additions and revisions to the nomenclature of specificities defined by both molecular and serological techniques following the principles established in previous reports (*1, 2, 3, 4, 5, 6, 7, 8, 9, 10, 11, 12, 13*).

The main subjects discussed were:
1. The naming of new genes within the HLA region
2. Naming of new alleles
3. Naming of alleles with altered levels of expression
4. Naming of serological specificities
5. Funding of the Nomenclature report and sequence database

1. The naming of new genes within the HLA region

Recently a number of new genes have been identified within the HLA region including some whose functions are related to HLA class I and II genes. The Committee discussed what its strategy should be for the naming of these and further new genes. It concluded that the naming of such genes raised many new issues and that, in order to name these genes appropriately it was desirable to co-opt onto the committee individuals with additional expertise in the structure and function of the new genes. We therefore decided to defer the naming of any new genes until the next meeting of the nomenclature committee.

2. Naming of new alleles

a. Conditions for acceptance of new allele sequences

As emphasized in previous reports, there are required conditions for acceptance of new sequences for official names.
1. Where a sequence is obtained from cDNA or where PCR products are subcloned prior to sequencing, several clones should have been sequenced.
2. If direct sequencing of PCR amplified material is performed, products from at least two separate PCR reactions should have been sequenced.
3. Sequencing should be performed in both directions.
4. Where possible a novel sequence should be confirmed by a DNA typing method such as PCR-SSOP or PCR-SSP.
5. An accession number in a databank should have been obtained.
6. Full length sequences are preferable though not essential; the minimum requirements are exons 2 and 3 for an HLA Class I sequence and exon 2 for an HLA Class II sequence.

* Address for correspondence: Dr Julia G. Bodmer, ICRF Cancer and Immunogenetics Laboratory, Institute of Molecular Medicine, John Radcliffe Hospital, Headington, Oxford OX3 9DU, UK, Tel. +44 1865 222361, Fax +44 1865 222384, e-mail: julia@icrf.icnet.uk

** New sequences should be communicated to Steven Marsh to receive official names. Address: Anthony Nolan Research Institute, Royal Free Hospital, Pond Street, Hampstead, London NW3 2QG, UK, Tel. +44 171 284-8321, Fax +44 171 284-8331, e-mail: marsh@icrf.icnet.uk

7. Where possible, a paper should have been submitted for publication.
8. DNA or other material, in particular cell lines, should be made available in a publicly accessible repository or at least in the originating laboratory. Documentation on this will be maintained by the Nomenclature Committee.
9. Submission of a sequence to the Nomenclature Committee should include a computer readable copy of the sequence. Researchers will be expected to complete a questionnaire relating to the sequence and provide a comparison of their new sequence with known related alleles.

It should be noted with some caution that cells from which only partial sequences have been obtained may later be shown to represent different or novel alleles when further sequencing is performed. This is of particular importance in cases where several different cells have been partially sequenced for an allele. In such cases, all cell lines have been listed in this report.

Official designations are currently being assigned to new alleles in the period between Nomenclature Committee meetings, provided they meet the criteria outlined above. Details of the newly reported alleles are published in monthly nomenclature updates in the journals Tissue Antigens, Human Immunology and the European Journal of Immunogenetics. The listing of references to new sequences does not imply priority of publication. The use of numbers or names for alleles, genes or specificities which pre-empt formal designations such as "HLA-M", "A*0103", "DRB5*0108" or "HLA-DL" before consideration by the Nomenclature Committee is strongly discouraged.

b. New Alleles

In the Class I region 27 HLA-A, 68 HLA-B, 12 HLA-C, one HLA-E and three HLA-G alleles were named, as shown in Tables 2, 3, and 4. The sequences of A*2412, A*3005, A*31011, A*3302, Cw*0101, Cw*0201, Cw*1201, Cw*1401, Cw*1501 and Cw*1603 have all been shown to be in error and these designations have been deleted. The cells originally sequenced for these alleles have now been shown to express respectively the A*2408, A*3004, A*31012, A*3303, Cw*0102, Cw* 02022, Cw*12022, Cw*1402, Cw*1502 and Cw* 1403 alleles (*24, 25, 141*) (K. Tokunaga and W. Hildebrand, personal communications). A complete listing of all the allele names which have now been deleted is given in Table 10.

In the Class II region 62 DRB1, seven DRB3, five DRB4, seven DRB5, two DQA1, six DQB1, two DPA1, 16 DPB1 and one DMB alleles were named. The sequences of DRB1*09011, DRB1*12031, DRB1*1606 and DPB1*02011 have all been shown to be in error and these designations have been deleted. The cells originally sequenced for these alleles have now been shown to express respectively the DRB1* 09012, DRB1*1201, DRB1*1605 and DPB1* 02012 alleles. Additionally, the DRB4 null allele previously named DRB4*0101102N has been shown to have been incorrectly assigned (*114*); this has now been corrected to DRB4*0103102N.

The name DRB1*1313 was first assigned in December 1993. The submitted sequence was consistent with it having been generated by motif shuffling or double recombination events as is commonly seen in newly reported alleles. However, shortly afterwards the authors retracted their sequence having shown it to be an error (*13*). Recently, a sequence was reported to the Nomenclature Committee that is identical to that originally designated DRB1*1313 (*C. Hurley, personal communication*), consequently this name has now been reinstated.

Many HLA sequences have only been reported by a single laboratory and from a single cell. In such cases, researchers are encouraged to submit confirmatory sequence reports to the Nomenclature Committee for inclusion in the HLA Sequence Database. They are also encouraged to submit cell lines which have been sequenced for novel HLA alleles for inclusion in the International Histocompatibility Workshop cell panel.

As discussed previously, with the continuing discovery of new HLA allele sequences, it is becoming increasingly difficult to maintain the link given by the allele name between the sequence and the serological profile of the antigen associated with it. In many cases, with researchers relying heavily on DNA technology they are unable to provide a serological definition, and where this is available, they often cannot place the newly defined antigen within a known serological grouping. This is especially true of the DRB1*03, *11, *13, *14 and *08 family of alleles and the description of new alleles within this group illustrates that this is in fact a continuum of allelic diversity. We would like to stress that, although it is our goal wherever possible to indicate the serological grouping into which an allele will fall, this is not always possible, and that most importantly the name should be seen as no more than a unique designation.

3. Naming of alleles with altered levels of expression

Previously an optional "N" was introduced to indicate a non-expressed or null allele. Recently, a novel

A*2402 allele has been reported by two groups (*P. Parham and M. Laforet, personal communications*) (*142*), where a mutation in a non-coding region has led to a significant decrease in the level of expression of the allele, it has therefore been decided to use an optional "L" to indicate alleles which are associated with unusual expression levels. Thus the normal A*2402 allele will become A*2402101 and the mutant allele with low cell surface expression will have the allele designation A*2402102L.

As discussed before, such extended allele names should only be used where it is clearly appropriate. In cases where it is not possible to define all the possible variations between alleles, a truncated allele designation is suggested. Thus if it is not possible to distinguish between the A*68011 and A*68012 alleles, the designation A*6801 is sufficient. Likewise, if it is not possible to discriminate between the twenty-two alleles encoding A2 then the designation A*02 is appropriate. In addition, DRB4*0103 is an alternative to DRB4*0103101, if this is not ambiguous in the context used.

4. Naming of serological specificities

Three new HLA Class I serological specificities were named: HLA-A80, -B2708 and -B81. Additionally, B7801, which was previously assigned (*11*), has now been shortened to B78 to take account of the second allele, B*7802, which is also found to be associated with this serological specificity.

New serological specificities have usually only been assigned following an International Histocompatibility Workshop. It has been decided to change this policy and discuss the naming of serological specificities on an annual basis. Since the most recent workshop did not include the exchange of a comprehensive set of HLA typing sera for serological analysis and it seems unlikely that this will form a part of any future workshop, it is our intention to work closely with the organisers of the International Cell Exchange co-ordinated by Paul Terasaki and Marie Lau in Los Angeles, to identify antigens which require official designations.

5. Funding of the Nomenclature report and sequence database

In September 1996 the HLA Sequence Database moved from the Imperial Cancer Research Fund, where it had been maintained since 1979, to the Anthony Nolan Research Institute (ANRI). It is proposed that the database will continue to be maintained at the ANRI for the foreseeable future, but we still urgently need to find a source of funding to support its continued maintenance. We are, therefore, currently discussing with users of the sequence database possible means of securing such support.

Acknowledgments

The committee would like to thank the Imperial Cancer Research Fund for its continued support. The support of Biotest for the committee meeting is also gratefully acknowledged.

List of committee members involved in preparing this report:

E. D. Albert, Policlinic for Children, University of Munich, Germany (Chairman)
J. G. Bodmer, Imperial Cancer Research Fund, Oxford, UK (Rapporteur)
S. G. E. Marsh, Anthony Nolan Research Institute, London, UK (Coordinator)
W. F. Bodmer, Imperial Cancer Research Fund, Oxford, UK
B. Dupont, Sloan-Kettering Institute for Cancer Research, New York, N.Y., USA
H. A. Erlich, Roche Molecular Systems, Alameda, Ca., USA
B. Mach, University of Geneva, Geneva, Switzerland
W. R. Mayr, University of Vienna, Vienna, Austria
P. Parham, Stanford University School of Medicine, Stanford, Ca., USA
T. Sasasuki, Kyushu University, Fukuoka, Japan
G. M. Th. Schreuder, University Hospital, Leiden, The Netherlands
J. L. Strominger, Harvard University, Cambridge, Ma., USA
A. Svejgaard, State University Hospital, Copenhagen, Denmark
P. I. Terasaki, University of California, Los Angeles, Ca., USA

Co-opted members:

R. E. Bontrop, Biomedical Primate Research Centre, Rijswijk, The Netherlands
D. C. Charron, Institut Biomédical des Cordeliers, Paris, France
R. Fauchet, Hopital Pontchaillou, Rennes, France

References

1. WHO Nomenclature Committee. *Bull. WHO* 1968: **39**: 483.
2. WHO Nomenclature Committee. WHO terminology report. In P.I. Terasaki ed. Histocompatibility Testing, 1970, Copenhagen: Munksgaard, 1970: 49.
3. WHO Nomenclature Committee. *Bull. WHO* 1972: **47**: 659.
4. WHO Nomenclature Committee. *Bull. WHO* 1975: **52**: 261.
5. WHO Nomenclature Committee. *Bull. WHO* 1978: **56**: 461.
6. WHO Nomenclature Committee. In PI Terasaki ed. Histocompatibility Testing, 1980, Los Angeles: UCLA Tissue Typing Laboratory, 1980: 18–20.
7. WHO Nomenclature Committee. Nomenclature for factors of the HLA system 1984. In ED Albert, MP Baur and WR Mayr eds. Histocompatibility Testing, 1984, Berlin: Springer-Verlag, 1985: 4–8.
8. Bodmer WF, Albert E, Bodmer JG, Dupont B, Mach B, Mayr WR, Sasazuki T, Schreuder GMT, Svejgaard A, Terasaki PI. Nomenclature for factors of the HLA system, 1987. In B. Dupont ed. Immunobiology of HLA, New York: Springer-Verlag, 1989: 72–79.
9. Bodmer JG, Marsh SGE, Parham P, Erlich HA, Albert E, Bodmer WF, Dupont B, Mach B, Mayr WR, Sasasuki T, Schreuder GMT, Strominger JL, Svejgaard A, Terasaki PI. Nomenclature for factors of the HLA system, 1989. *Tissue Antigens* 1990: **35**: 1–8.
10. Bodmer JG, Marsh SGE, Albert E, Bodmer WF, Dupont B, Erlich HA, Mach B, Mayr WR, Parham P, Sasasuki T, Schreuder GMT, Strominger JL, Svejgaard A, Terasaki PI. Nomenclature for factors of the HLA system, 1990. *Tissue Antigens* 1991: **37**: 97–104.
11. Bodmer JG, Marsh SGE, Albert E, Bodmer WF, Dupont B, Erlich HA, Mach B, Mayr WR, Parham P, Sasasuki T, Schreuder GMT, Strominger JL, Svejgaard A, Terasaki PI. Nomenclature for factors of the HLA system, 1991. In T Tsuji, M Aizawa and T Sasazuki eds. HLA 1991, Oxford: Oxford University Press, 1992: 17–31.
12. Bodmer JG, Marsh SGE, Albert E, Bodmer WF, Dupont B, Erlich HA, Mach B, Mayr WR, Parham P, Sasasuki T, Schreuder GMT, Strominger JL, Svejgaard A, Terasaki PI. Nomenclature for factors of the HLA system, 1994. *Tissue Antigens* 1994: **44**: 1–18.
13. Bodmer JG, Marsh SGE, Albert E, Bodmer WF, Bontrop RE, Charron D, Dupont B, Erlich HA, Mach B, Mayr WR, Parham P, Sasasuki T, Schreuder GMT, Strominger JL, Svejgaard A, Terasaki PI. Nomenclature for factors of the HLA system, 1995. *Tissue Antigens* 1995: **46**: 1–18.
14. Dale Y, Kimura A, Kato H, Sasazuki T. DNA typing of the HLA-A gene: population study and identification of four new alleles in Japanese. *Tissue Antigens* 1996: **47**: 93–101.
15. Kashiwase K, Ishikawa Y, Tokunaga K, Ohashi H, Hashimoto M, Lin L, Akaza T, Tadokoro K, Juji T. Sequence of a new HLA-A allele (A*0218) encoding a serological variant, HLA-A2K, observed in Japanese. *Tissue Antigens* 1996: **48**: 329–330.
16. Fleischhauer K, Zino E, Mazzi B, Severini GM, Benazzi E, Bordignon C. HLA-A*02 subtype distribution in caucasians from northern Italy: identification of A*0220. *Tissue Antigens* 1996: **48**: 673–679.
17. Szmania S, Gasque-Carter P, Baxter-Lowe L-A. Nucleotide sequence for A*0221 which encodes a novel HLA Class I polymorphic residue. *Tissue Antigens* 1996: **48**: 720–724.
18. Liernert K, Russ G, Lester S, Bennett G, Gao X, McCluskey J. Stable inheritance of an HLA-A "blank" phenotype associated with a structural mutation on the HLA-A*0301 gene. *Tissue Antigens* 1996: **48**: 187–191.
19. Bettinotti MP, Mitsuishi Y, Lau M, Silver H, Spence A, Terasaki PI. HLA-A*1104: a new allele found in a Laotian family. *Tissue Antigens* 1996: **48**: 717–719.
20. Gao X, Matheson B. A novel HLA-A*24 (A*2410) allele identified in a Javanese population. *Tissue Antigens* 1996: **48**: 711–713.
21. Maruya E, Ishikawa Y, Lin L, Tokunaga K, Kimura A, Nita H, Yokoyama, S., Saji H. Allele typing of HLA-A10 group by nested-PCR-low ionic strength single stranded conformational polymorphism and a novel A26 allele (A26KY, A*2605). *Human Immunology* 1996: **50**: 140–147.
22. Arnett KL, Moses JM, Williams F, Marsh SGE, Bodmer JG, Parham P, Middleton D. HLA-A*2607: Sequence of a novel A*26 subtype predicted by DNA typing which shares the MA2.1 epitope with A*02, B*57 and B*58. *Tissue Antigens* 1996: **47**: 422–425.
23. Szmania S, Baxter-Lowe LA. Nucleotide sequence of a novel HLA-A26 gene encoding glutamine at codon 156. *Tissue Antigens* 1996: **48**: 210–212.
24. Blasczyk R, Wehling J, Päßler M, Hahn U, Huhn D, Salama A. A novel HLA-A30 allele (A*3004) identified by single-strand conformation polymorphism and confirmed by solid-phase sequencing. *Tissue Antigens* 1995: **46**: 322–326.
25. Arnett KL, Adams EJ, Parham P. On the sequence of A*3101. *Tissue Antigens* 1996: **47**: 428–430.
26. Zino E, Severini GM, Mazzi B, Bordignon C, Benazzi E, Fleischhauer K. Sequencing of a new subtype of HLA-A*32. *Immunogenetics* 1996: **45**: 76–77.
27. Binder T, Wehling J, Huhn D, Blasczyk R. Increased diversity within the HLA-A*66 group: Implications for matching in unrelated bone marrow transplantation. *Tissue Antigens* 1997: **50**: 77–82
28. Blasczyk R, Wehling J, Önaldi-Mohr D, Rebmann V, Chandanayingyong D, Grosse-Wilde H. Structural definition of the A*74 group: Implications for matching in bone marrow transplantation with alternative donors. *Tissue Antigens* 1996: **48**: 205–209.
29. Smith KD, Epperson DF, Lutz CT. Alloreactive cytotoxic T-lymphocyte-defined HLA-B7 subtypes differ in peptide antigen presentation. *Immunogenetics* 1995: **43**: 27–37.
30. Sanz L, Vilches C, de Pablo R, Moreno ME, Kreisler M. Haplotypic association of two new HLA class I alleles: Cw*15052 and B*0706. Evolutionary relationships of

HLA-Cw*15 alleles. *Tissue Antigens* 1996: **47**: 329–333.

31. Grundschober C, Rufer N, Adami N, Breur-Vriesendorp B, Jeannet M, Roosnek E, Tiercy J-M. Sequence of a new HLA-B7 variant, B*0707, that differs from the common B*0707 allele by one single residue in the peptide binding groove. *Tissue Antigens* 1997: **49**: 508–511
32. Eberle M, Lorentzen D, Iwanaga KK, Hennes LF, Watkins DI. Identification of a new HLA-B*08 variant, HLA-B*0804. *Tissue Antigens* 1997: **49**: 256–261
33. Lin L, Tokunaga K, Nakajima F, Ishikawa Y, Kashiwase K, Tanaka H, Kuwata S, Sideltseva EW, Akaza H, Tadokorro K, Shibata Y, Chandanayingyong D, Juji T. Both HLA-B*1301 and B*1302 exist in Asian populations and are associated with different haplotypes. *Human Immunology* 1995: **43**: 510–56.
34. Lin L, Tokunaga K, Tanaka H, Nakajima F, Imanishi T, Kashiwase K, Bannai M, Mizuno S, Akaza T, Tadokoro K, Shibata Y, Juji T. Further molecular diversity in the HLA-B15 group. *Tissue Antigens* 1996: **47**: 265–274.
35. Hurley CK, Steiner N, Hoyer RJ, Menchaca E, Mitton W, Simonis T, Hartzman RJ, Johnson AH, Ng J. Novel HLA-B alleles, B*8201, B*3515, and B*5106, add to the complexity of serologic identification of HLA types. *Tissue Antigens* 1996: **47**: 179–187.
36. Martinez-Laso J, Layrisse Z, Gomez-Casade E, Montova F, Guédez Y, Dominguez E, Varela P, Arnaiz-Villena A. A new HLA-B15 allele (B*1522) found in Bari-Motilones Amerindians in Venezuela: comparison of its intron 2 sequence with those of B*1501 and B*3504. *Immunogenetics* 1995: **43**: 108–109.
37. Cereb N, Kim C, Hughes AL, Yang SY. Molecular analysis of HLA-B35 alleles and their relationship to HLA-B15 alleles. *Tissue Antigens* 1997: **49**: 389–396
38. Curran MD, Williams F, Middleton D. A novel HLA-B allele, HLA-B*1803. *Tissue Antigens* 1996: **48**: 708–710.
39. Rudwaleit M, Bowness P, Wordsworth P. The nucleotide sequence of HLA-B*2704 reveals a new amino acid substitution in exon 4 which is also present in HLA-B*2706. *Immunogenetics* 1996: **43**: 160–162.
40. Hasegawa T, Ogawa A, Sugahara Y, Moriyama Y, Nanzai H, Tawara K, Tokunaga K, Juji T, Kondo S. Novel HLA-B27 allele (B*2711) encoding an antigen reacting with both B27 and B40 specific antisera. *Tissue Antigens* 1997: **49**: 649–652
41. Adams EJ, Little A-M, Arnett KL, McAuley JE, Williams RC, Parham P. Three new HLA-B alleles found in Mexican-Americans. *Tissue Antigens* 1995: **46**: 414–416.
42. Curran MD, Williams F, Middleton D. Long range PCR amplification as an alternative strategy to characterising novel HLA-B alleles. *Eur. J. Immunogenetics* 1996: **23**: 297–309.
43. Vargas-Alarcón G, Martinez-Laso J, Granados J, Diaz-Campos N, Alvarez M, Gomez-Casado E, Alcocer-Varela J, Arnaiz-Villena A. Description of a novel HLA-B35 (B*3514) allele found in a Mexican family of Nahua Aztec descent. *Human Immunology* 1996: **45**: 148–151.
44. Vargas-Alarcón G, Alvarez M, Martinez-Laso J, Granados J, Diaz-Campos N, Gomez-Casado E, Alcocer-Varela J, Arnaiz-Villena A. A new HLA-B35 (B*3516) allele found in a Mexican of Nahua (Aztec) descent. *Immunogenetics* 1996: **43**: 244–245.
45. Vargas-Alarcón G, Martinez-Laso J, Gomez-Casado E, Granados J, Diaz-Campos N, Varela P, Alvarez M, Arnaiz-Villena A. A novel HLA-B35 (B*3517) allele found in a Mexican of Otomi ascent. *Tissue Antigens* 1996: **47**: 547–550.
46. Santos S, Vicario JL, Merino JL, Balas A. Characterization of a new HLA-B allele (B*3702) generated by an intronic recombination event. *Immunogenetics* 1996: **43**: 171–172.
47. Zhao W, Fernandez-Viña MA, Lazaro AM, Araujo HA, Miller S, Stastny P. Full cDNA of a novel HLA-B39 subtype, B*39061. *Tissue Antigens* 1996: **47**: 435–437.
48. Garber TL, McAdam SN, Butler LM, Crocker P, Piekarczyk M, Troup GM, Milford EL, Watkins DI. HLA-B alleles of the Navajo: no evidence for rapid evolution in the Nadene. *Tissue Antigens* 1996: **47**: 143–146.
49. Ramos M, Postigo JM, Vilches CV, Layrisse Z, López de Castro JA. Primary structure of a novel HLA-B39 allele (B*3909) from the Warao Indians of Venezuela. Further evidence for local HLA-B diversification in South America. *Tissue Antigens* 1995: **46**: 401–404.
50. Wells RS, Parham P. A novel recombinant HLA-B*39 allele (B*3910) in a South African Zulu. *Tissue Antigens* 1996: **48**: 595–597.
51. Vilches C, Bunce M, de Pablo R, Moreno ME, Puente S, Sanz L, Kreisler M. A novel HLA-Cw*1802-B*5703 haplotype detected in the Bubi population from Equatorial Guinea. *Tissue Antigens* 1997:**49**: 644–648
52. Adams EJ, Little A-M, Arnett K, Leuschner J, Parham P. Identification of a novel HLA-B40 allele (B*4008) in a patient with Leukemia. *Tissue Antigens* 1995: **46**: 204–205.
53. Ando H, Mizuki N, Ohno S, Tabbara KF, Taguchi S, Yamazaki M, Mizuki N, Miyata Y, Wakisaka K, Inoko H. Identification of a novel HLA-B allele (B*4202) in a Saudi Arabian family with Behçet's disease. *Tissue Antigens* 1997: **49**: 526–528
54. Zhao W, Fernandez-Viña MA, Lazaro AM, Araujo HA, Miller S, Stastny P. Complete cDNA sequence of B*4406, an HLA-B allele containing sequences of B*5101 and B*4402. *Tissue Antigens* 1996: **47**: 431–434.
55. Vilches C, Sanz L, de Pablo R, Moreno ME, Puente S, Kreisler M. Molecular characterisation of the new alleles HLA-B*8101 and B*4407. *Tissue Antigens* 1996: **47**: 139–142.
56. Fischer GF, Broer E, Faé I, Leitner D, Mayr WR. Nucleotide sequence analysis of an HLA-B47 variant (HLA-B*4702). *Tissue Antigens* 1997: **49**: 540–542
57. Prillman K, Steiner N, Ellexson M, Stewart D, Lau M, Terasaki P, Hurley C, Hildebrand W. Novel alleles HLA-B*7802 and B*51022: Evidence for convergence in the HLA-B5 family. *Tissue Antigens* 1996: **47**: 49–57.
58. Curran MD, Williams F, Rima BK, Markwick J, Middleton D. A new HLA-B51 allele, B*5107 in RCE55 detected and characterised by PCR-SSOP, cloning and nu-

cleotide sequence determination. *Tissue Antigens* 1996: **48**: 228–230.
59. Williams F, Curran MD, Vaughan RW, Page G, Middleton D. Identification of a new HLA-B*55 allele, HLA-B*5503. *Tissue Antigens* 1996: **48**: 598–599.
60. Bannai M, Tokunaga K, Tanaka H, Lin L, Kashiwase K, Tokunaga K, Juji T. Five HLA-B22 group alleles in Japanese. *Tissue Antigens* 1997: **49**: 376–382
61. Szmania S, Seurynck K, Baxter-Lowe L-A. Nucleotide sequence of HLA-B*5505 which expresses a unique HLA class I polymorphism. *Tissue Antigens* 1997: **49**: 537–539
62. Barnardo MCNM, Bunce M, Lord CJ, Welsh KI. HLA-B*5603: Sequence of a novel hybrid allele comprising B*56 and B*4601. *Tissue Antigens* 1997: **49**: 496–498
63. Andrien M, Defleur V, De Canck I, Bouillenne C, Jannes GR, R. and Dupont, E. B*78022, a new Caucasian member within the B78 family. *Tissue Antigens* 1997: **49**: 79–83.
64. Ellexson M, Stewart D, Chretien P, Zhang L, Hildebrand W. A modified sequencing strategy for the molecular characterization of HLA-B*8201. *Tissue Antigens* 1996: **47**: 438–441.
65. Wang H, Tokunaga K, Akaza T, Tadokoro K, Shibata Y, Juji T. Identification of HLA-C alleles using PCR-single stranded-conformation polymorphism and direct sequencing. *Tissue Antigens* 1997: **49**:134–140
66. Zarling A, Smith KD, Lutz CT, Lee DR. Correction of the HLA-Cw3 genomic sequence tentatively identifies it as HLA-Cw*0304. *Immunogenetics* 1996: **44**: 82–83.
67. Little A-M, Mason A, Marsh SGE, Parham P. HLA-C typing of eleven Papua New Guineans: Identification of an HLA-Cw4/Cw2 hybrid allele. *Tissue Antigens* 1996: **48**: 113–117.
68. Wang H, Tokunaga K, Ishikawa Y, Asahina A, Kuwata S, Akaza T, Tadokoro K, Shibata Y, Takiguchi M, Juji T. Identification and DNA typing of two Cw7 alleles (Cw*0702 and Cw*0704) in Japanese, with the corrected sequence of Cw*0702. *Human Immunology* 1996: **45**: 52–58.
69. Vilches C, Bunce M, Sanz L, de Pablo R, Puente S, Kreisler M. Molecular cloning of two new HLA-C alleles: Cw*1801 and Cw*0706. *Tissue Antigens* 1996: **48**: 698–702.
70. Wang H, Tokunaga K, Ogawa A, Akaza T, Tadokoro K, Takiguchi MS, Shibata, Y., Juji T. DNA typing of Cw14 alleles in Japanese and the corrected sequence of Cw*1402. *Tissue Antigens* 1996: **47**: 442–446.
71. Cereb N, Hughes AL, Yang SY. Cw*1701, a new HLA-C allelic lineage with an unusual transmembrane domain. *Tissue Antigens* 1997: **49**: 252–255
72. Herrero MJ, Vilches C, de Pablo R, Puente S, Kreisler M. The complete primary structure of Cw*1701 reveals a highly divergent HLA class I molecule. *Tissue Antigens* 1997: **49**: 267–270
73. Wang H, Tokunaga K, Akaza T, Shibata Y, Juji T. A novel allele, Cw*1702 with serological Cw2 specificity. *Tissue Antigens* 1997: **49**: 183–185.
74. Yamashita T, Fujii T, Watanabe Y, Tokunaga K, Tadokoro K, Juji T, Taketani Y. HLA-G gene polymorphism in a Japanese population. *Immunogenetics* 1996: **44**: 186–191.
75. Morales P, Corell A, Martinez-Laso J, Martín-Villa JM, Varela P, Paz-Artal E, Allende L-M, Arnaiz-Villena A. Three new HLA-G alleles and their linkage disequilibria with HLA-A. *Immunogenetics* 1993: **38**: 323–331.
76. Yamashita T, Fujii T, Tokunaga K, Tadokoro K, Juji T, Taketani Y. Correction of the HLA-G*01012 genomic sequence. *Tissue Antigens* 1997: **49**: 673–674
77. Hashemi S, Couture C, Buyse I, Cole R, Aye MT. Identification of a new DRB1*13 (DRB1*1320) and a novel DRB1*15 allele (DRB1*15012) with a silent mutation affecting oligotyping. *Tissue Antigens* 1996: **47**: 147–149.
78. Wu S, Yabe T, Madden M, Saunders TL, Bach FH. cDNA cloning and sequencing reveals that the electrophoretically constant DR β2 molecules, as well as the variable DR β1 molecules, from HLA-DR2 subtypes have different amino acid sequences including a hypervariable region for a functionally important epitope. *J. Immunology* 1987: **138**: 2953- 2959.
79. Fei H, Lu Y, Lin B, Jiang W, Zou Y, Chen R. The nucleotide sequence of a new HLA DR15(2) allele in Chinese. *Chinese Journal of Microbiology & Immunology* 1995: **15**: 45–48.
80. Shinno K, Tsuboyama K, Mine H, Maruya E, Nita H, Masuda H, Yamagata N, Tsuji H, Nakagawa M, Saji H. Nucleotide sequence of a new DRB1*15 variant, 1505, in a Japanese family. *Tissue Antigens* 1995: **46**: 411–413.
81. van den Berg-Loonen EM, Rani R, Singal D, Tilanus M. A new DRB1*15 allele (DRB1*1506) identified by sequence based typing. *Tissue Antigens* 1997: **49**: 189–191.
82. White JM, Baxter-Lowe LA. Sequence of DRB1*1601. *Tissue Antigens* 1997: **49**: 192–193.
83. Trejaut J, Bhatia K, Greville WD, Hu KR, Duraisamy G, Nuchprayoon C, Donald J, Aziz A, Dunckley H. HLA-DR2 haplotypic diversity in four populations of Southeast Asia and Northern China, and five Melanesian populations using PCR-RFLP for DRB1, DRB5, DQB1 and DQA1. A new DRB1 allele. *Eur. J. Immunogenetics* 1996: **23**: 437–449.
84. Anholts JDH, Bouwens AGM, Verduyn W, Tilanus MGJ, Schreuder GMT. Sequence of HLA-DRB1*1606 is incorrect. *Human Immunology* 1996: **46**: 65–66.
85. Israel S, Smith AG, Marashi A, Hansen JA, Brautbar C. Two new DR2 alleles; DRB1*1607 identified in a Ashkenazi Jewish family and DRB1*15022 found in a single caucasian donor. *Tissue Antigens* 1997: **49**: 171–173
86. Ellis JM, Steiner N, Wang J, Tang T, Hurley CK. Diversity and evolution of the DRB1*03 family: Description of DRB1*03022, *0307, *0308. *Tissue Antigens* 1997: **49**: 41–45.
87. Fenske B, Lemieux J, Hoar D, Fitzpatrick J, Keown P. A novel DRB1*0306 allele identified by PCR-RFLP. *Human Immunology* 1996: **46**: 55–57.
88. Dufossé F, Guignier F, Cracco P, Becuwe D, Huart J-J. A novel HLA DRB1 allele (DRB1*0309). *Tissue Antigens* 1997:**49**: 523–525
89. Martinez-Quiles N, Martin-Villa JM, Martinez-Laso J,

Ferre-Lopez S, Moreno-Pelayo MA, Alvarez-Tejado M, Arnaiz-Villena A. Description of two new DRB1 (DRB1* 0310) and DRB3 (DRB3*01012) alleles found in a Spanish infant. *Tissue Antigens* 1997: **49**: 658–666
90. Thonnard J, Gervais T, Heusterpreute M, Mersch G, De Canck I, De Greef C, Demanet C, Van Waeyenberge C. A new silent mutation at codon 35 in exon 2 yielding DRB1*04012 allele. *Tissue Antigens* 1997: **49**: 274–277
91. Moribe T, Kaneshige T, Hirakata M, Mimori T, Akitsuki M, Inoko H. Identification of a DRB1*0405 variant (DRB1* 04052) using the PCR-RFLP method. *Tissue Antigens* 1996: **47**: 450–453.
92. Gebuhrer L, Adami N, Javaux F, Freidel AC, Jeannet M, Betuel H, Tiercy J-M. Sequence of a new HLA-DR4 allele with an unusual residue at position 88 that does not seem to affect T-cell allo recognition. *Human Immunology* 1996: **51**: 60–62.
93. Murru MR, Costa G, Murru R, Muntoni F, Marrosu MG. A new allelic variant of HLA-DRB1*1101 (DRB1* 11013) segregating in a Sardinian family. *Tissue Antigens* 1996: **48**: 604–606.
94. Heron SD, McKeen ME, Cizman BB, Kerans DJ, Argyris EG, Wu J, Griffith BB, Kamoun M, Zmijewski CM, Bunin N, Monos DS, Williams TM. Identification of HLA-DRB1*1114 by oligonucleotide typing and DNA sequencing. *Immunogenetics* 1995: **42**: 436–437.
95. Nielsen J, Zhang G, Spalding T, Cao K, Hunter J, Chopek M. Molecular cloning and automated sequencing of a new HLA-DRB1 allele within the DRB1*14 family. *Human Immunology* 1995: **44–1**: 52.
96. Smith AG, Nelson JL, Regen L, Guthrie LA, Donadi E, Mickelson EM, Hansen JA. Six new DR52-associated DRB1 alleles, three DR8, two DR11, and one of DR6 reflect a variety of mechanisms which generate polymorphism in the MHC. *Tissue Antigens* 1996: **48**: 118–126.
97. Cizman BB, Kearns DJ, McKeen ME, Heron SD, Wu J, Griffith BB, Argyris EG, Kamoun M, Zmijewski CM, Williams TM, Monos DS. New DRB1*1120 allele; another example of the transition between the DR11 and DR13 families of alleles. *Tissue Antigens* 1996: **48**: 52–54.
98. Verduyn W, Anholts JDH, Versluis LF, Parlevliet J, Drabbels J, De Meester J, Tilanus MGJ, Doxiadis IIN, Giphart MJ, Schreuder GMT. Six newly identified HLA-DRB alleles: DRB1*1121, *1419, *1420, *1421, DRB3*0203 and DRB5*0103. *Tissue Antigens* 1996: **48**: 80–86.
99. Adami N, Jeannet M, Tiercy J-M. Sequence of a new HLA-DR11 allele with a DR4-specific first hypervariable region. *Immunogenetics* 1995: **42**: 448–449.
100. Schranz P, Seelig R, Seidl C, Renz M. Nucleotide sequence of a new HLA-DRB1*11 allele (DRB1*1124). *Immunogenetics* 1996: **43**: 242–243.
101. Perrier P, Reveillere C, Schuhmacher A. A new DRB1 allele (DRB1*1125) sharing DR11 and DR8 sequence motifs. *Tissue Antigens* 1997: **49**: 84–87.
102. Knipper AJ, Enczmann J, Schuch B, Uhrberg M, Kögler G, Wernet P. A novel HLA-DRB1*11 allele (DRB1* 1127). *Tissue Antigens* 1997: **49**: 414–416
103. Rodriguez SG, Crevling CL, Steiner N, Hurley CK. Identification of a new allele, DRB1*1204, during routine PCR-SSOP typing of National Marrow Donor Program volunteers. *Tissue Antigens* 1996: **48**: 221–223.
104. Cizman BB, Heron SD, McKeen ME, Kearns DJ, Bassinger S, Griffith BB, Argyris EG, Kamoun M, Zmijewski CM, Williams TM, Monos DS. Identification of DRB1 allele (DRB1*1316) with aspartate at position 86: Evolutionary considerations and functional implications. *Tissue Antigens* 1996: **47**: 153–154.
105. Dormoy A, Delbosc A, Galy-Floc'h M, Tongio M. A novel DRB1*13 allele (DRB1*1318) with a short DR B1*08 sequence. *Immunogenetics* 1996: **43**: 240–241.
106. Poli F, Bianchi P, Crespiatico L, Sirchia G. Identification of a new DRB1 allele (DRB1*1325) by PCR-SSP and DNA sequencing. *Tissue Antigens* 1996: **48**: 714–716.
107. Voorter CEM, de Bruyn-Geraets D, Verduyn W, Schreuder GMT, van den Berg-Loonen EM. Identification of a new HLA-DRB1*13 allele (DRB1*1326) with a short DRB1* 16 sequence. *Tissue Antigens* 1997: **49**: 88–91.
108. Schaffer M, Olerup O. A novel DRB1*13 allele (DRB1* 1327) on a DR17, DQ2 haplotype with a DRB1*0301 sequence motif in the second hyperpolymorphic region. *Tissue Antigens* 1997: **49**: 186–188.
109. Löffler D, Wölpl A, Kern P, Eiermann TH. A novel HLA-DR allele, DRB1*1419. *Tissue Antigens* 1995: **46**: 343–344.
110. Adami N, Aubert V, Jeannet M, Tiercy JM. Sequencing of a new HLA-DR14 allele (DRB1*1422). *Immunogenetics* 1996: **43**: 248–249.
111. Kashiwase K, Tokunaga K, Lin L, Sugahara N, Miyamoto M, Akaza T, Tadokoro K, Juji T. A new HLA-DR8 subtype showing unusual serological reaction and the confirmatory sequence of DRB1*0809. *Tissue Antigens* 1995: **46**: 340–342.
112. Versluis LF, Savelkoul PHM, van der Zwan A-W, van den Berg-Loonen EM, Tilanus MGJ. Identification of the new HLA-DRB1*0812 allele detected by sequencing based typing. *Immunogenetics* 1996: **43**: 169–170.
113. Trejaut J, Greville W, Duncan N, Dunckley H. A novel allele (DRB1*0815) defined in an Australian Aborigine. *Tissue Antigens* 1997: **49**: 529–531
114. Naruse TK, Ando R, Nose Y, Kagiya M, Ando H, Kawata H, Nabeya N, Isshiki G, Inoko H. HLA-DRB4 genotyping by PCR-RFLP: diversity in the association between HLA-DRB4 and DRB1 alleles. *Tissue Antigens* 1997: **49**: 152–157
115. De Canck I, Demant C, Mersch G, Jannes G, Rombout A, Rossau R, Van Waeyenberge C. Characterization of a new DRB4 allele (DRB4*0104). *Tissue Antigens* 1996: **48**: 213–216.
116. Voorter CEM, Emonds M-P, van den Berg-Loonen EM. Identification of a new DRB4 allele (DRB4*0105) by sequence-based-typing. *Tissue Antigens* 1997: **49**: 662–664
117. Poli F, Bianchi P, Crespiatico L, Terragna C, Sirchia G. Characterisation of a new HLA-DRB5 allele (DRB5* 0105) by PCR-SSP and direct sequencing. *Tissue Antigens* 1996: **47**: 338–340.

118. Freeman SM, Saunders TL, Madden M, Segall M, Bach FH, Wu S. Comparison of DRβ1 alleles from diabetic and normal individuals. *Human Immunology* 1987: **19**: 1–6.

119. Yasunaga S, Kimura A, Hamaguchi K, Rϕnningen KS, Sasazuki T. Different contribution of HLA-DR and -DQ genes in susceptibility and resistance to Insulin-dependant Diabetes Mellitus (IDDM). *Tissue Antigens* 1996: **47**: 37–48.

120. Lee KW, Johnson AH, Hurley CK. New DQw1 diversity identified within DRw12 and DRw14 haplotypes. *Tissue Antigens* 1991: **38**: 231–234.

121. Schranz P, Nessler G, Schindera F, Seelig R. Nucleotide sequence of the corrected DQB1*06011 allele. *Tissue Antigens* 1996: **48**: 139–140.

122. Mersch G, Sémana G, De Canck I, Jannes G, Sterker G, Rossau R. Characterization of a new DQB1 allele (DQB1*0610) which differs from DQB1*0602 at the highly polymorphic 57-codon. *Tissue Antigens* 1996: **48**: 217–220.

123. Williams TM, Bassinger S, Moehlenkamp C, Wu J, Montoya GD, Griffith BB, McAuley JD, Goldman S, Maurer DH, Troup GM. Strategy for distinguishing a new DQB1 allele (DQB1*0611) from the closely related DQB1*0602 allele via sequence specific PCR or direct DNA sequencing. *Tissue Antigens* 1996: **48**: 143–147.

124. Vilches C, García-Pacheco J-M, de Pablo R, Puente S, Kreisler M. Complete coding region of the new HLA-DQB1*0612 allele, obtained by RT-PCR. *Tissue Antigens* 1996: **48**: 589–592.

125. Trachtenberg EA, Keyeux G, Bernal J, Nobel J, Erlich HA. Results of Expedicion Humana. II. Analysis of HLA class II alleles in three African American populations from Colombia using the PCR/SSOP: Identification of a novel DQB1*02 (*0203) allele. *Tissue Antigens* 1996: **48**: 192–198.

126. Olerup O, Aldener-Cannavá A, Fogdell-Hahn A, Getty RR, Wagenknecht DR, McIntyre JA. DQB1*0202 and the new DQB1*0203 allele: A fourth pair of DQB1 alleles only differing at codon 57. *Tissue Antigens* 1997: **49**: 271–273

127. Saito S, Ota S, Hashizume K, Kaneshige T, Kinoshita T, Hashimoto M, Oguchi H, Ishii E, Yamada E. A new HLA-DQB1*0306 allele sharing DQB1*03032 and DQB1*04 sequences. *Tissue Antigens* 1996: **48**: 580–585.

128. Thye T, Muntau B, Stelma FE, Horstmann RD. Novel allele DQB1*0307 in a West African family. *Tissue Antigens* 1997: **49**: 517–518

129. May J, Kretschmer C, Schnittger L, Striecker R, Kremsner PG, Meyer CG. DPA1*0105, a novel DPA1 – variant in a negroid population. *Tissue Antigens* 1996: **48**: 593–594.

130. Muntau B, Thye T, Pirmez C, Horstmann RD. A novel DPA1 allele (*0203) composed of known epitopes. *Tissue Antigens* 1997: **49**: 668–669

131. Schranz P, Renz M, Wojtzyk I, Seelig R. Nucleotide sequence of a new HLA-DPB1 allele, DPB1*02013. *Immunogenetics* 1996: **44**: 159–160.

132. Noble JA, Cavalli AS, Erlich HA. DPB1*5901: A novel HLA-DPB1 allele from a Caucasian family with insulin-dependant diabetes mellitus. *Tissue Antigens* 1996: **47**: 159–162.

133. Noreen H, Steiner L, Davidson M, Johnson S, Segall M, Begovich AB. Six new DPB1 alleles identified in a study of 1,302 unrelated bone marrow donor-recipient pairs. *Tissue Antigens* 1997: **49**: 512–516

134. Zimmerman PA, Steiner LL, Titanji VPK, Nde PN, Bradley JE, Pogonka T, Begovich AB. Three new DPB1 alleles identified in a Bantu-speaking population from central Cameroon. *Tissue Antigens* 1996: **47**: 293–299.

135. Steiner LL, McCurdy DK, Cavalli A, Moonsamy PV, Begovich AB. Two new DPB1 alleles identified in a study of the genetics of susceptibility to pauciarticular juvenille rheumatoid arthritis. *Tissue Antigens* 1997: **49**: 262–266

136. Versluis LF, Phillipe M, Van der Zwan A, Thonnard J, Tongio MM, Tilanus MGJ. Identification of a new HLA-DPB1*6501 allele in a Caucasian individual. *Immunogenetics* 1996: **44**: 483–484.

137. Schnittger L, May J, Kretschmer C, Kremsner PG, Meyer CG. DPB1*BR – an Mhc class II DPB1 allele (DPB1* 6601) of negroid origin. *Immunogenetics* 1996: **44**: 405–406.

138. Meyer CG, May J, Simon C, Boehm BO, Loeliger C-C. DPB1*TF, a novel HLA class II DPB1 allele identified in a Turkish family. *Tissue Antigens* 1996: **48**: 231–232.

139. Naruse TK, Kawata H, Ishihara M, Ando A, Kagiya M, Nose Y, Isshiki G, Inoko H. Analysis on allelic variation of the HLA-DMB gene in Japanese by PCR-RFLP as well as direct DNA sequencing and identification of a new DMB allele, DMB*0105. *Tissue Antigens* 1996: **47**: 530–537.

140. Kim T-G, Carrington M, Choi H-B, Kim H-Y, Han H. Three HLA-DMB variants in Korean patients with autoimmune diseases. *Human Immunology* 1996: **46**: 58–60.

141. Bunce M, Barnardo MCNM, Procter J, Marsh SGE, Vilches C, Welsh KI. High resolution HLA-C typing by PCR-SSP: identification of allelic frequencies and linkage disequilibria in 604 consecutive unrelated random UK Caucasians and a comparison with serology. *Tissue Antigens* 1996: **48**: 680–691.

142. Parham P. Definition and importance of HLA class I null alleles: a new role for serological HLA class I typing. In D. Charron ed. Genetic Diveristy of HLA: Functional and Medical Implications, Volume 2, Sevres: EDK, 1997: pp. 28–34.

TABLE 1. Names for genes in the HLA region.

Name	Previous equivalents	Molecular characteristics
HLA-A	–	Class I α-chain
HLA-B	–	Class I α-chain
HLA-C	–	Class I α-chain
HLA-E	E, '6.2'	associated with class I 6.2-kB Hind III fragment
HLA-F	F, '5.4'	associated with class I 5.4-kB Hind III fragment
HLA-G	G, '6.0'	associated with class I 6.0-kB Hind III fragment
HLA-H	H, AR, '12.4'	Class I pseudogene associated with 5.4-kB Hind III fragment
HLA-J	cda12	Class I pseudogene associated with 5.9-kB Hind III fragment
HLA-K	HLA-70	Class I pseudogene associated with 7.0-kB Hind III fragment
HLA-L	HLA-92	Class I pseudogene associated with 9.2-kB Hind III fragment
HLA-DRA	DRα	DR α chain
HLA-DRB1	DRβI, DR1B	DR β1 chain determining specificities DR1, DR2, DR3, DR4, DR5 etc.
HLA-DRB2	DRβII	pseudogene with DR β-like sequences
HLA-DRB3	DRβIII, DR3B	DR β3 chain determining DR52 and Dw24, Dw25, Dw26 specificities
HLA-DRB4	DRβIV, DR4B	DR β4 chain determining DR53
HLA-DRB5	DRβIII	DR β5 chain determining DR51
HLA-DRB6	DRBX, DRBs	DRB pseudogene found on DR1, DR2 and DR10 haplotypes.
HLA-DRB7	DRBψ1	DRB pseudogene found on DR4, DR7 and DR9 haplotypes.
HLA-DRB8	DRBψ2	DRB pseudogene found on DR4, DR7 and DR9 haplotypes.
HLA-DRB9	M4.2 β exon	DRB pseudogene, isolated fragment
HLA-DQA1	DQα1, DQ1A	DQ α chain as expressed
HLA-DQB1	DQβ1, DQ1B	DQ β chain as expressed
HLA-DQA2	DXα, DQ2A	DQ α-chain-related sequence, not known to be expressed
HLA-DQB2	DXβ, DQ2B	DQ β-chain-related sequence, not known to be expressed
HLA-DQB3	DVβ, DQB3	DQ β-chain-related sequence, not known to be expressed
HLA-DOB	DOβ	DO β chain
HLA-DMA	RING6	DM α chain
HLA-DMB	RING7	DM β chain
HLA-DNA	DZα, DOα	DN α chain
HLA-DPA1	DPα1, DP1A	DP α chain as expressed
HLA-DPB1	DPβ1, DP1B	DP β chain as expressed
HLA-DPA2	DPα2, DP2A	DP α-chain-related pseudogene
HLA-DPB2	DPβ2, DP2B	DP β-chain-related pseudogene
TAP1	RING4, Y3, PSF1	ABC (ATP Binding Cassette) transporter
TAP2	RING11, Y1, PSF2	ABC (ATP Binding Cassette) transporter
LMP2	RING12	Proteasome-related sequence
LMP7	RING10	Proteasome-related sequence

TABLE 2. Designations of HLA-A alleles.

HLA Alleles[a]	HLA Specificity	Previous Equivalents	Individual or Cell Line from which the Sequence was Derived	Accession Number	References or Submitting Author(s)
A*0101	A1	–	LCL721, MOLT4, PP	X55710, M24043	
A*0102	A1	–	DAUDI	U07161	
A*0201	A2	A2.1	LCL721, JY, GM637, GRC138, T5-1, JD	M32322, K02883, M84379, X02457	
A*0202	A2	A2.2F	M7, 951314	M17566, M17568, X94566	R. Blasczyk[b]
A*0203	A203	A2.3	DK1, 951315	U03863, M17567, M19670, X94567	R. Blasczyk[b]
A*0204	A2	–	RML, AN, 951316	X57954, M86404, X94568	R. Blasczyk[b]
A*0205	A2	A2.2Y	WT49, AM, SUS-NF, 951317	U03862, L76290, X94569	P. Parham[b], R. Blasczyk[b]
A*0206	A2	A2.4a	CLA, T7526, 951318	M24042, X94570	R. Blasczyk[b]
A*0207	A2	A2.4b	KNE, KTO	D50458	K. Tokunaga[b]
A*0208	A2	A2.4c	KLO	X94571	R. Blasczyk[b]
A*0209	A2	A2-OZB	OZB	–	
A*0210	A210	A2-LEE	XLI-ND, 951322	Z23071, X94572	R. Blasczyk[b]
A*0211	A2	A2.5	KIME, GRC138, 951366	X60764, M84377, X94573	R. Blasczyk[b]
A*0212	A2	–	KRC033, KRC005	M84378	
A*0213	A2	A2SLU	SLUGEO	Z27120	
A*0214	A2	A2'1S'	1S	Z30341	
A*0215N	A'Blank'	HLA-Anull	TSU	D38525	
A*0216	A2	A2'TUB'	TUBO	Z46633	
A*0217	A2	A*New	AMALA, LZL, C.S.	U18930, L43526, L43527, X89707, X89708	(14)[b], R. Blasczyk[b]
A*0218	A2	A*2K	ENDO	D83515	(15)
A*0219	–	A-02X09	TOB-81	L76936	P. Stastny
A*0220	A2	–	BI	X96724	(16)
A*0221	A2	A206W331R	W331R	U56825	(17)
A*0222	A2	A-02x28	TER-109	U76398, U76399	P. Stastny
A*0301	A3	A3.1	JG, JD, PP, AP630	X00492, K02057, U32184	W. Hildebrand[c]
A*0302	A3	A3.2	E1B2, R69772	U56434, U56435	C. Hurley[b]
A*0303N	A'Blank'	A3blank	MMK	L77702	(18)
A*1101	A11	A11E, A11.1	CJO-A, K.LIE, MMU, YMU	M16007, M16008, X13111, D16841	
A*1102	A11	A11K, A11.2	K.LIE, KOK, CTA	X13112, D16842	
A*1103	A11	–	AMAD	X91399	H. Tijssen
A*1104	A11	–	HM, I65	U50574, U59701, U59702	(19), D. Bugawan
A*2301	A23(9)	–	SHJO, ELON	M64742, L76288	P. Parham[b]
A*2402101[d]	A24(9)	A24, A2402	SHJO, 32/37, KRC032, KRC110	M64740, M84376, L47206, Z72423	P. Parham[b], M. Laforet[b]
A*2402102L	–	A2402LOW, APET	6319, PAn, PMa, PMi	L76291, Z72422	P. Parham, M. Laforet
A*2403	A2403	A9.3	APA, KPE	M64741	
A*2404	A24(9)	A24AK	ITOU, KJRAID5	D26550, L43532, L43533	(14)[b]

HLA Alleles[a]	HLA Specificity	Previous Equivalents	Individual or Cell Line from which the Sequence was Derived	Accession Number	References or Submitting Author(s)
A*2405	A24(9)	A24New	DST, FST	X82161, X82189	
A*2406	A24(9)	A*24YM	YM29	U18987, U19733	
A*2407	A24(9)	A#46	PICH, A#46, K92068	U25971, U36914, L43530, L43531	(14), A. Selvakumar, M. Chopek
A*2408	A24(9)	A*9HH	K62098, HIRH	L43528, L43529, D83516	(14), K. Tokunaga
A*2409N	A'Blank'	A24Null	SUS-NF	L47231	P. Parham
A*2410	A9	A*24JV	JV1458, KM315	U37110, U37111, U59699, U59700	(20), D. Bugawan
A*2411N	A'Blank'	A*24LM	LUME	L76289	P. Parham
A*2413	A24(9)	A*24YM2	YM81	U37112, U37113	X. Gao
A*2414	A24(9)	A*24SA	SBD6380	U37114, U37115	X. Gao
A*2501	A25(10)	–	BM92	M32321	
A*2502	A10	A66var	M54672	X97802	P. Krausa
A*2601	A26(10)	A26.1, A26.3	GM637, O2BN5, MGAR, N.M., MIY-2, MIY-3	M24095, U03697, D16843, D32130, D32131	
A*2602	A26(10)	A26.2, A26.1	KT14, Y.I., E.K.	M98453, D14350	
A*2603	A26(10)	A26.4	T.M., S.M., MIY-1	D14351, D32129	
A*2604	A26(10)	A10SA	Y.S.	D14354	
A*2605	A26(10)	A26KY	SAJ022, K91089, K93022	D50068, L43536, L43537	(14, 21)
A*2606	A26(10)	–	KHB102	L43534, L43535	(14)
A*2607	A26(10)	A26mic	MIC-ND	L48341	(22)
A*2608	A26(10)	A26RMH	MI108, W652D, M.McL	U45480, U52429, X99733	(23), W. Hildebrand, D. Middleton
A*2901	A29(19)	–	JOE	M23739	
A*2902	A29(19)	A29.2	LAM	X60108	
A*2903	–	–	CMD004AN	Y09218	A-M. Little
A*3001	A30(19)	A30.3, A30RSH	LBF, RSH	M30576, M28414, U07234	
A*3002	A30(19)	A30.2	CR-B	X61702	
A*3003	A30(19)	A30JS	JS, HT	M93657	
A*3004	A30(19)	A*30AD, A30W7, A30JW	AD7563, W7(CC), ASE	U18988, U19734, Z34921, X83770, X83771	(24)[c]
A*31012	A31(19)	–	KRC033, TB, KRC110, JHAF, KT12	M30578, M28416, M84375, M86405, L78918	(25)[c]
A*3201	A32(19)	–	AM	P10314	
A*3202	A32(19)	–	MP	X97120	(26)
A*3301	A33(19)	Aw33.1	JOE, LWAGS, LCL80	M30580, M28415, U18989, U19735, X83004-5	
A*3303	A33(19)	A33NC, A33MK	CTM4955926, GAO801, LCL82, HOR, IT	U09740, U18990, U19736, X83002-3, L06440	
A*3401	A34(10)	–	ENA	X61704	
A*3402	A34(10)	–	WWAI	X61705	
A*3601	A36	–	MASCH	X61700	
A*4301	A43	–	CC	X61703	
A*6601	A66(10)	–	25/1506, TEM, GU5175	X61711, U17571	

HLA Alleles[a]	HLA Specificity	Previous Equivalents	Individual or Cell Line from which the Sequence was Derived	Accession Number	References or Submitting Author(s)
A*6602	A66(10)	–	CR-B, MALS, HUT102	X61712, X51745	
A*6603	A10	A66KA	AKI	X96638	(27)
A*68011	A68(28)	Aw68.1	LB	X03070, X03071	
A*68012	A68(28)	Aw68.1	GRC187	L06425	
A*6802	A68(28)	Aw68.2	PA, TO	U03861	
A*6803	A28	–	AA859, PIME	U41057, U56436, U56437	W. Hildebrand, C. Hurley
A*6901	A69(28)	–	IDF, ZM, BJ	X03158, X03159	
A*7401	A74(19)	–	CC, PDAV, ATUR, GU2037, GU2040	X61701, U17569, U17570	
A*7402	A74(19)	A*74dc	DCH-HLA05	X95409	(28)
A*7403	A19	A*74pb	PEB	X95561	(28)
A*8001	A80	AX"BG", A-new	VH, 35020, 35841, 32511, CODI, MIKA, LADA, CTM3953540, CTM1953541	M94880, L18898, L19403, U03754	

[a]Allele names given in bold type have been assigned since the 1995 Nomenclature report.
[b]This reference is to a confirmatory sequence.
[c]This reference is to a corrected sequence.
[d]This sequence has been previously assigned with a four digit allele name.

TABLE 3. Designations of HLA-B alleles.

HLA Alleles[a]	HLA Specificity	Previous Equivalents	Individual or Cell Line from which the Sequence was Derived	Accession Number	References or Submitting Author(s)
B*0702	B7	B7.2, B*07L	JY, PP, RD105U, RD105, L5, L7, GN00105	M16102, M32317, M35444, P01889, U29057, L47338, U49904, U49905	W. Hildebrand[b], A. Arnaiz-Villena[b], C. Hurley[b]
B*0703	B703	BPOT	POT71, BPot	X64454, U21053	(29)[b]
B*0704	B7	B7E	10243	U04245	
B*0705	B7	B*07ZEL	GEE018, ZEL, CF	L33922, U18661, U21052	(29)[b]
B*0706	B7	B7-L79	L7901	X91749	(30)
B*0707	B7	–	DAPO	Z70315	(31)
B*0708	–	–	A.McG	X99735	D. Middleton
B*0801	B8	–	LCL721, MF, CGM1, HECO	M59841, M24036, M28204, L76093	P. Stastny[b]
B*0802	B8	B8JON, B8V	20015, 19315	U04244	
B*0803	B8	B*O8NR	NR	U28759	E. Petersdorf
B*0804	–	B*08New-UW	BLB, JS, PF	U67330, U67331, U74386	(32), C. Hurley
B*1301	B13	B13.1	HE, SDI, YTY, TAC	M24075, D50290	(33)[b]
B*1302	B13	B13.2, B13N	LBF, TO, HJB, PKM, TAC	M19757, M24041, D50291	(33)[b]
B*1303	–	B New	CTM4956865, CTM2956866	U14943	
B*1304	–	B*15X21	TER847	U75533	W. Hildebrand
B*1401	B64(14)	–	MRWC, 32367, W6106, WT51	M24040, X94574	R. Blasczyk[b]
B*1402	B65(14)	–	BB, CGM1	M59840, M24032	
B*1501	B62(15)	–	MF, HA, BCK, OLGA (OLL)[d], KT17, PP, FUR, YAG, BA3, BA4, BA5	M28203, M83193, U03859, D50292, L48400	(34)[b], A. Arnaiz-Villena[b]

HLA Alleles[a]	HLA Specificity	Previous Equivalents	Individual or Cell Line from which the Sequence was Derived	Accession Number	References or Submitting Author(s)
B*1502	B75(15)	B15N	APA, LW, CAY	M75138, M83192, D50293	(34)[b]
B*1503	B72(70)	–	CC, 26931, 31708	X61709	
B*1504	B62(15)	Bw62-G	GRC138, KG, GRC187	M84382, M86402	
B*1505	B62(15)	Bw62.1	VB	M83191	
B*1506	B62(15)	Bw62.4	WI	M83194	
B*1507	B62(15)	Bw62.5	SB	M83195	
B*1508	B62(15)	B62variant	KHAGNI, LATIF, DAN723	L11666	
B*1509	B70	B70.1	34863	L11571	
B*1510	B71(70)	B70.2	25514, 19014, GU373, GU2092, GU2037, GU5175	L11570, U11262, U11264, U11269	
B*1511	B15	B15variant, B75v	LEE743, AZ195, AZ319	L11604, D50294	(34)[b]
B*1512	B76(15)	B76	THAI742	L11603	
B*1513	B77(15)	B77	RSA-ND, CAM020, PETCH	L15005, D50295	(34)[b]
B*1514	B76(15)	B76	SS713	L19937	
B*1515	B62(15)	B62s	MLH727, LDM	L22027, L49343	A. Arnaiz-Villena[b]
B*1516	B63(15)	B63.1, 8W66	DOP-ND, 21909, 31133	L09735	
B*1517	B63(15)	B63	JAP-NF, PARMG	U01848, U35431	(35)[b]
B*1518	B71(70)	B*7901, B"X"-HS, B71	HS, GU2739, GU2760, MSU, ML108, ML108U	U11266, U11268, D50296, U57966	(34)[b], W. Hildebrand[b]
B*1519	B76(15)	B76	GEE018	U03027	
B*1520	B62(15)	–	OLGA (OLL)[d], KRC110	U06862	
B*1521	B75(15)	B15Ab	BJ, HWY, 14247373	L32862, D44500, U32678	(34)[b], C. Hurley[b]
B*1522	–	B15UW1, B35V2	1274, B503, JC (G2997)	U14756, L42506, U34619	(36, 37)[b]
B*1523	–	B'NM5'	TK765	L37881	
B*1524	B62(15)	B*15ZEL, 1501-B4a, B*1501-Bw4	ZEL, SF94-140	U16309, L42146	P. Stastny[b]
B*1525	B62(15)	B*15AOH	WON, M, HM, BY0007	U18660, U50710, U52177, U52178	(19)[b], C. Hurley[b]
B*1526N	B'Blank'	B-null	K.I.	D49824	H. Mine
B*1527	B62(15)	–	PELE	L42144, L40182	P. Stastny
B*1528	B15	B15v1	YTR	D44499	(34)
B*1529	B15	B15v3	DKA	D44501	(34)
B*1530	B75(15)	B*1501V1	EFTO, GN00104, GN00108	L42296, U49900, U49901, U52171, U52172	P. Stastny, C. Hurley
B*1531	B75(15)	B*1502V	ALDE, GN00110	L42145, U52173, U52174	P. Stastny, C. Hurley
B*1532	B62(15)	–	DCH036	X95410	R. Blasczyk
B*1533	B15	–	GN00103	U49898, U49899	C. Hurley
B*1534	B15	–	GN00105	U49902, U49903	C. Hurley
B*1535	B15	–	GN00106	U52167, U52168	C. Hurley
B*1536	–	B*15MD	MD674	U58315, U58316	X. Gao
B*1537	–	–	11112331	U55022, U55023	C. Hurley
B*1801	B18	–	SGAR, F24	M24039	

HLA Alleles[a]	HLA Specificity	Previous Equivalents	Individual or Cell Line from which the Sequence was Derived	Accession Number	References or Submitting Author(s)
B*1802	B18	B18PE	PETCH	D25275	
B*1803	B18	–	BM66, GSW002	X94480, Y07824	(38), R. Blasczyk
B*1804	–	B*18IM	IMM348	U38792, U38793	X. Gao
B*1805	B18	B*18GSW	GSW001	Y07710	
B*2701	B27	27f	LH, PIL-139	L76935	P. Stastny[b]
B*2702	B27	27e, 27K, B27.2	BRUG, NV, KSH	X03664, X03667, L38504, U18659	
B*2703	B27	27d, 27J	CH (CHI)[d]	M54883, M37272	
B*2704	B27	27b, 27C, B27.3	WEWAK 1, DH, DEW-ND	U27608	(39)[b]
B*27052	B27	27a, 27W, B27.1	CD, HC, MRWC, KCA, MVL, LG2, BRUG	X03945, M12967, L20086, M14013, M12678	
B*27053	B27	B27MW	HHE	X83727, X83737	
B*2706	B27	27D, B27.4	LIE, PAR	X73578, U35734	(39)[b]
B*2707	B27	B27-HS	HS	M62852	
B*2708	B2708	B7Qui	19418, BCK	L19923	
B*2709	B27	B27-ci	Ci	Z33453	
B*2710	B27	B2705v	KRICO	L76095	P. Stastny
B*2711	B27	B27KH	K.H.	D83043	(40)
B*3501	B35	–	HS, KT17, GU2739, CMM	M28109-12, U11265, L63544	A. Arnaiz-Villena[b]
B*3502	B35	–	DL	M63454	
B*3503	B35	–	C1R, HMY2, 12405, 13159	M81798, D50299	K. Tokunaga[b]
B*3504	B35	–	AN, RB22, 12.36JK	M86403, U30936, L47986	W. Hildebrand[b], A. Arnaiz-Villena[b]
B*3505	B35	B35-G	GRC212, KRC032, TOB-115	M84385, L76930	P. Stastny[b]
B*3506	B35	B35-K	KRC032	M84381	
B*3507	B35	–	#20073	L04695	
B*3508	B35	B35TL	#22338, TL	L04696, Z22651	
B*35091[c]	B35	–	MA9	U17107	
B*35092	B35	–	WIC-54	L76932	P. Stastny
B*3510	–	–	JK1.2, JK5.13, JK14.41	L36979	
B*3511	B35	B35v	GRC-187	L40599	P. Parham
B*3512	B35	B-3504v	BAON, FEME, PNS	L42281, L76094, L49342	(41), P. Stastny, A. Arnaiz-Villena
B*3513	B35	2993	RCE80	X87268	(42)
B*3514	B35	B*35M	JLG, JGS	L42545	(43)
B*3515	B35	–	PARMG	U30904	(35)
B*3516	–	B*35GAR	GAR	U29880	(44)
B*3517	B35	B35V1, B*35PNS, B-3505v	JM (G2744), PNS, AMYE	U34618, L49341, L75941	(37, 45), P. Stastny
B*3518	B35	B-3508v	TOB-137	L75942	P. Stastny
B*3519	B35	B-40X35	WIC-54	L76933	P. Stastny
B*3520	B35	B-3501V	TER-135	U76392, U76393	P. Stastny
B*3521	–	B-3511H	TER-109	U76390, U76391	P. Stastny
B*3701	B37	–	KAS011, MG, GU2760	M32320, U11267	
B*3702	–	B27-37	CTM-8958127	U31971	(46)

HLA Alleles[a]	HLA Specificity	Previous Equivalents	Individual or Cell Line from which the Sequence was Derived	Accession Number	References or Submitting Author(s)
B*3801	B38(16)	B16.1	Z, JAP-NF, YAR, JBUSH, TEM, WDV, ELON, LB96-SAR	M29864, L36591, U40498	V. Brichard[b]
B*3802	B38(16)	–	RSA-ND	L22028	
B*39011	B3901	B39.1, B16.2	S, JC	M94052, M29865	
B*39013	B3901	B39.1J	IT, #591	M94051	
B*39021	B3902	B39.2	YAM	M94053	
B*39022	B3902	B39.2	CL170	U04243	
B*3903	B39(16)	–	AUCA#19	L20088	
B*3904	B39(16)	B39N	TO	L22649	
B*3905	B16	ST-16, B*39UW1, B*39JAI	11, HGOM, 12.35JK, 12.63JK	U15638, L36318, L36980	A. Arnaiz-Villena[b]
B*39061	B39(16)	B*39UW2	15, HAA, BA1, TER-102	U15639, L42024, L76640, L76639, U76396, U76397	(47)[b], A. Arnaiz-Villena[b], P. Stastny[b]
B*39062	B39(16)	B*39DBU, B39G	DBU, GVA, CVL, RD105, NAVAJO	U16298, L40562, U29083, U32660	(48)[b], A. Arnaiz-Villena[b], W. Hildebrand[b]
B*3907	–	B*39UW3	1276	U15640	
B*3908	B39(16)	–	822	L42280	(41)
B*3909	B39(16)	B39-143.2	143.2, XAV-50	U29480, L76088	(49), P. Stastny
B*3910	B39(16)	B39.ZU47	Zu47, GN00110, GB32	U56246, U52175, U52176, Y09058	(50, 51), C. Hurley
B*3911	–	–	KUNA 20	U74387	M. Eberle
B*3912	B39(16)	B-3901V	TER-103	U76394, U76395	P. Stastny
B*40011	B60(40)	–	LB	P01890, U03698	
B*40012	B60(40)	B60Ut	Ut-m, JD, #W7079	M95530, L41628	
B*4002	B61(40)	B40*	SWEIG, CALOGERO, YUKI, 19014, TOB-105	L09736, D14343, L76089	P. Stastny[b]
B*4003	B40	B40-G1	GRC138	M84383	
B*4004	B40	B40-G2	GRC212, TOB-0087	M84384, L76090	P. Stastny[b]
B*4005	B4005	BN21	00136	M84694	
B*4006	B61(40)	B61	Ot-s	M95531	
B*4007	–	B'Fu'	MSU, FTA, KTA	D31816	
B***4008**	–	–	4008	L41353	(52)
B*4009	B61(40)	B-4003V	PIL-117	L76934	P. Stastny
B*4010	B60(40)	B*40MD	MD676	U58643, U58644	X. Gao
B*4101	B41	–	SGAR	M24035	
B*4102	B41	B41.2	SBD4, GU5175, BM2684	X81363, U17572, X86704	(42)[b]
B*4201	B42	–	BB	M24034	
B***4202**	B42	B42ANDO	E-117, E-119	D50709	(53)
B*4402	B44(12)	B44.1, B44.2	FMB, BAU	M24038, M15470	
B***44031**[c]	B44(12)	B44.1:New	PITOUT, F24	X64366	
B***44032**	B44(12)	–	OBH, SHCHA	L42282, U58469, U58470	(41), C. Hurley
B*4404	B44(12)	B44.4	TAN, BEB	X75953, X78426, X78427	
B*4405	B44(12)	B44WJG, B44KB	WJG, KB	X78849, X78850, L31798	

HLA Alleles[a]	HLA Specificity	Previous Equivalents	Individual or Cell Line from which the Sequence was Derived	Accession Number	References or Submitting Author(s)
B*4406	B44(12)	–	GIJM, KARY	X83400, X83401-3, L42345	(54)[b]
B*4407	B44(12)	B*44GB	GB92	X90391	(55)
B*4408	B44(12)	B44bo	19662	U64801	P. Parham
B*4409	B12	–	S.A.	X99734	D. Middleton
B*4410	–	–	S32	U63559, U63560	C. Hurley
B*4501	B45(12)	–	OMW	X61710	
B*4601	B46	–	T7527, THAI742	M24033	
B*4701	B47	–	PLH	M19756	
B***4702**	B47	–	CAL	Y09118	(56)
B*4801	B48	–	KRC103, HS67	M84380	
B*4802	B48	–	AUCA#18	L20089	
B***4803**	–	B-48.3	TOB-115	L76931	P. Stastny
B*4901	B49(21)	–	AM, GU2092	M24037, U11263	
B*5001	B50(21)	–	SH.JO, JD, GU2037	X61706, U11261	
B***5002**	–	B*50IM, B*45v	IMM754, WM1366C	U58317, U58318, Y08995	X. Gao, C. Vilches
B*51011[c]	B51(5)	–	LKT-2, TO, BM92, CD, LCL721, KRC110, KRC005, BA1, BA6	M32319, M21035, M22786-8, M28205, Z46808, L47985	A. Arnaiz-Villena[b]
B*51012	B51(5)	–	GN00106	U52169, U52170	C. Hurley
B*51021[c]	B5102	B5.35	UM, 02627	M68964	
B***51022**	B5102	–	MY823	L41925	(57)
B*5103	B5103	BTA	30-BY3	M80670	
B*5104	B51(5)	–	GRC150	Z15143	
B*5105	B51(5)	B51v	LK	U06697	
B*5106	B5	–	GN097, GN088	U31334, U32661	(35)
B*5107	B51(5)	B5101v	RCE55	X94481	(58)
B*5108	B51(5)	B*51FA, B*51GAC	F.A., GN00109, NDS-DG	X96473, U52815, U52816, Y08994	R. Blasczyk, C. Hurley, C. Vilches
B*5109	B51(5)	B*51IM	IMM721, NMDP-0004	U58319, U58320, U76400, U76401	X. Gao, P. Stastny
B*52011	B52(5)	–	MT, LK707	M21036, M22793-9	
B*52012	B52(5)	–	AUCA#2, TOB-137, BA8	L20090, L76091, L47984	P. Stastny[b], A. Arnaiz-Villena[b]
B*5301	B53	–	AMAI, AM	M33574, M58636	
B***5302**	–	–	S15(28)	U63561, U63562	C. Hurley
B*5401	B54(22)	–	LKT-3, TTL	M77774	
B*5501	B55(22)	–	VEN	M77778	
B*5502	B55(22)	–	APA	M77777	
B***5503**	–	B5501v	RCE70	X94482	(59)
B*5504	B55(22)	B-4201v, B55.2	TAGO, 11840Kane	L76225, D85761	(60), P. Stastny
B*5505	B22	B5501 W669R	B55W669R	U63653	(61)
B*5601	B56(22)	–	VOO	M77776	
B*5602	B56(22)	–	ENA	M77775	
B***5603**	B22	B22N, B56/46	15630Naka, 01300, 01094, NPC-4	D85762, U67746, U67747, U67749, U73113	(60, 62), C. Hurley

HLA Alleles[a]	HLA Specificity	Previous Equivalents	Individual or Cell Line from which the Sequence was Derived	Accession Number	References or Submitting Author(s)
B*5701	B57(17)	–	WIN, MOC, MOLT4	X55711, M32318	
B*5702	B57(17)	Bw57.2	32/32	X61707	
B*5703	B57(17)	B*57SAU	SAU, MAME, GB32	U18790, U39088, Y09157	(35, 51)[b]
B*5704	B57(17)	B-5702v	OPOU	L76096	P. Stastny
B*5801	B58(17)	–	WT49, DAUDI, GN00107, 1075011	M11799, U52813, U52814, U65395, U65396	C. Hurley[b]
B*5802	–	B58v	DAUDI, RCE56	L33923, X86703	(42)[b]
B*5901	B59	–	AT, KY, MAS	L07743, D50300	K. Tokunaga[b]
B*67011	B67	–	HS67, #591, #W7079, PVR	L17005, L76252	A. Arnaiz-Villena[b]
B*67012	B67	B*67LAV	LAV	U18789	
B*7301	B73	–	LK707, LE023, HL	U04787, X77658, L24373	
B*7801	B78	B'SNA',Bx1	SNA, 32/32	X61708, M33573	
B***78021**	B78	–	RC654	L41214	(57)
B*78022	B78	B78Hen	Hen	X96534, X96533	(63)
B*8101	B81	B'DT', B*7x48GB, B56b	AP630, GB92, 56B	L37880, X90390, U34810	(55)[b], M. Chopek[b]
B*8201	–	B22x45	MAME, MAMA, MAPA, RB22, VWAR	U29241, U38800, U36492	(35, 64)

[a]Allele names given in bold type have been assigned since the 1995 Nomenclature report.
[b]This reference is to a confirmatory sequence.
[c]This sequence has been previously assigned with a four digit allele name.
[d]Cell line is also known by alternative name.

TABLE 4. Designations of HLA-C, -E, -G alleles.

HLA Alleles[a]	HLA Specificity	Previous Equivalents	Individual or Cell Line from which the Sequence was Derived	Accession Number	References or Submitting Author(s)
Cw*0102	Cw1	Cw1.2, C1J1	T7527, AP, LCL721, KRC005, TTY, BRUG	M84171, Z46809, D50852, M16272	(65)[b]
Cw*0103	Cw1	C1J2	ITOU	D64145	K. Tokunaga
Cw*02021	Cw2	Cw2.2	MVL	M24030	
Cw*02022	Cw2	Cw2.2	SWEIG, BDG, BRUG	M26712, D83029, M16273	K. Tokunaga[b]
Cw*02023	Cw2	–	KACD	Z72007	J-M. Tiercy
Cw*0302	Cw10(w3)	–	AP, JG	M84172	
Cw*0303	Cw9(w3)	C3J1	GRC150, SJK	M99390, D50853	(65)[b]
Cw*0304	Cw10(w3)	C3J2	KRC110, JD, SKA, JG	M99389, D64150, U44064, U31372, U31373	(65, 66)[b]
Cw*0401	Cw4	C4J1	C1R, KSE	M84386, X58536, D83030	(65)[b]
Cw*0402	Cw4	BeWo C.1	BeWo	M26432	
Cw*0403	–	Cw4NM	KWO010	L54059	(67)
Cw*0501	Cw5	Cw5N	QBL, RC, JME, QBL	M58630, M34290, L24491, D64148, D83742	(65)[b]

HLA Alleles[a]	HLA Specificity	Previous Equivalents	Individual or Cell Line from which the Sequence was Derived	Accession Number	References or Submitting Author(s)
Cw*0602	Cw6	Cw6(W), C6J1	MS, G088, DJS, JOE, JD, TTU	M28206, X70857, Z22752-4, M28160, D64147	(65)[b]
Cw*0701	Cw7	–	MF, LCL721	M28207, Z46810	
Cw*0702	Cw7	JY328, Cw7J1, Cw7.5	JY, TID, KOK, WEHO	D38526, Z49112	J-M. Tiercy[b]
Cw*0703	Cw7	HLA-4	?	M11886	
Cw*0704	Cw7	Cw7/8v	LB33-MEL, KRO3/4, SSA, 40C	U09853, X83394, D49552, U38976	(68)[b], M. Chopek[b]
Cw*0705	–	39C	39C	U38975	M. Chopek
Cw*0706	Cw7	Cw*07GB	GB92	X97321	(69)
Cw*0707	–	Cw7v	HAUP	Z79751	J-M. Tiercy
Cw*0801	Cw8	C8J1	02627, KNM, SFK, HTS	M84174, D64151	(65)[b]
Cw*0802	Cw8	–	CGM1, LWAGS, WT51	M59865, M84173	
Cw*0803	Cw8	C8J2	KRC103, SSK	Z15144, D50854	(65)[b]
Cw*12021	–	Cb-2	MT	M28172, M28174, M28176, M28178	
Cw*12022	–	Cw*1202gyp, C12J1	G085, MSU, AKIBA	X70856, D64152, D83741, M21963, D12471-2	(65)[b]
Cw*1203	–	Cw12New, C12J12	D0208915, WDV, YAR, GB002, HNT	U06695, U06696, X82122, D64146	(65)[b]
Cw*1204	–	Sy/9-2	M.H(9-2)	X99704	Z. Tatari
Cw*1301	–	CwBL18	TCC	M58631, M34291	
Cw*1402	–	Cw14New	LUY, TC106, LKT2	U06487, Z47377, U41386, D49820, M28171, M28173, M28175, M28177	(70)[d], W. Hildebrand[b]
Cw*1403	–	Cx44	TID	D31817	W. Hildebrand
Cw*1502	–	C*X, Cw*6.2, Cl.9, Cw15J1	AUCA#2, G085, G088, KUE, GM637	L20091, X67818, D83031, M24096	(65)[b]
Cw*1503	–	–	GRC150	M99388	
Cw*1504	–	Cw*15Sp	C047	X73518	
Cw*15051[c]	–	Cw*15v	LE023	X78343	
Cw*15052	–	Cw*1505v	L7901	X87841	(30)
Cw*1601	–	Cl.10	GM637, TC106	M24097, U41420, U56259, U56260	W. Hildebrand[d], M. Chopek[d]
Cw*1602	–	Cw*16v	C073	X76189	
Cw*1604	–	Cw*16New	BOJ	Z75172	J-M. Tiercy
Cw*1701	–	Cw16New	RSH, GB86	U06835, X98742	(71, 72)[d], P. Parham[d]
Cw*1702	–	Cw17N	KSU	D64149	(73)
Cw*1801	–	Cw*04GB, Cw4x6	GB92, DIJL	X96582, Z80227	(69), J-M. Tiercy
Cw*1802	–	Cw*18GB	GB32	Y09156	(51)
E*0101	–	JTW15	JT, YN, HF, SPAARN70	M20022, L78934	A. Arnaiz-Villena[b]
E*0102	–	HLA-6.2	LCL721	M21533	
E*01031[c]	–	M32507, E*01C230	MT, MH, TK, SPAARN70, CHI009, JFE	M32507, L78455, X87678, X87679, L78455	A. Arnaiz-Villena[b], R. Blasczyk[b]

HLA Alleles[a]	HLA Specificity	Previous Equivalents	Individual or Cell Line from which the Sequence was Derived	Accession Number	References or Submitting Author(s)
E*01032	–	E*01T230	MSC, CHI004, 17771	X87680, X87681, L79943	R. Blasczyk, A. Arnaiz-Villena
E*0104	–	M32508	KS	M32508	
G*01011	–	HLA-6.0, G*I	LCL721.144, ASR53, MOU, SPO010, YRK	J03027, X17273, L27836, L27837, D77998, D77999, D78000	(74)[b]
G*01012	–	BeWo G7, G*II, GJ2	BeWo, COX, DHIF, WT47, YRK	M32800, X60983, Z14154, L41392, D85032, D67009, D67010, D67011	(74, 75, 76)[d]
G*01013	–	G*IV, GJ4	BeWo, KKH	L07784, L20777, L41363, D67003-5, D85033	(74, 75)
G*0102	b 150	Ice 6.23-5.4H	ICE 6	S69897	
G*0103	b 150	G*III	LWAGS	M99048	
G*0104	–	GJ3	YRK, CHI525	D67006, D67007, D67008, L78072	(74), A. Arnaiz-Villena
G*0105N	–	G*1.5	DCH027	L78073	A. Arnaiz-Villena

[a]Allele names given in bold type have been assigned since the 1995 Nomenclature report.
[b]This reference is to a confirmatory sequence.
[c]This sequence has been previously assigned with a four digit allele name.
[d]This reference is to a corrected sequence.

TABLE 5. Designations of HLA-DR alleles.

HLA Alleles[a]	HLA-DR Serological Specificities	HLA-D-Associated (T-cell-defined) Specificities	Previous Equivalents	Individual or Cell Line from which the Sequence was Derived	Accession Number	References or Submitting Author(s)
DRA*0101	–	–	DRα, PDR-α-2	JY, RAJI, F.G.	J00194, J00196, J00203	
DRA*0102	–	–	DR-H	JY	J00201	
DRB1*0101	DR1	Dw1	–	45.1, LG2	X03069, M11161	
DRB1*01021[c]	DR1	Dw20	DR1-NASC	NASC, 1568	–	
DRB1*01022	DR1	Dw20	DRB1*01DMT	TO0973	Z50871	S. Hashemi
DRB1*0103	DR103	Dw'BON'	DR1-CETUS, DRB1*BON	RAI, BG, BON	M33600	
DRB1*0104	DR1	–	DRB1*01New	L.R.	X70261	
DRB1*15011[c]	DR15(2)	Dw2	DR2B Dw2	PGF, ROF-NL	M17378, M16957, M20430	
DRB1*15012	DR15(2)	Dw2	DRB1*15MT	LD0797	Z48359	(77)
DRB1*15021	DR15(2)	Dw12	DR2B Dw12	BGE, DHO	M16958, M30180, M28584	(78)[b]
DRB1*15022	DR15(2)	Dw12	DR2MU	CMURD	L23964	
DRB1*1503	DR15(2)	–	–	G247	M35159	
DRB1*1504	DR15(2)	–	DR2DAI	D13, D53, HM	L23963, L34025	(79)[b]

HLA Alleles[a]	HLA-DR Serological Specificities	HLA-D-Associated (T-cell-defined) Specificities	Previous Equivalents	Individual or Cell Line from which the Sequence was Derived	Accession Number	References or Submitting Author(s)
DRB1*1505	DR15(2)	–	DRB1*15KY	K.W.	D49823	(80)
DRB1*1506	DR15(2)	–	–	JB317836, RP, CANSIN009, INDRAN001, INDRAN003	D63586, U45999, X98256	(81), N. Nagao, D. Sese
DRB1*16011[c]	DR16(2)	Dw21	DR2B Dw21	AZH, MN-2, FJO, W692D, W738D	M16959, M30179, M28583, U56640	(78, 82)[f]
DRB1*16012	DR16(2)	Dw21	–	GN00150	U59686	C. Hurley
DRB1*16021[c]	DR16(2)	Dw22	DR2B Dw22	REM (RML)[d]	M20504	
DRB1*16022	DR16(2)	Dw22	DRB1*16MADANG	MAD009	U38520	(83)
DRB1*1603	–	–	–	JWR	L02545	
DRB1*1604	DR16(2)	–	DRB1*16x8	BONA, FORE	L14852	
DRB1*1605	DR2	–	16PRET	EH.B., PRET4149	X74343, X75444	(84)[f]
DRB1*1607	–	–	DR2Mut	USH	U26659	(85)
DRB1*1608	–	–	DRB1*(Gi+Pi)	Gi, Pi	Z72424	A. Dormoy
DRB1*03011	DR17(3)	Dw3	–	RAJI, AVL, WT49, DM24, DM28, DM29, CMCC	M17379, X04054	
DRB1*03012	DR17(3)	Dw3	DRB1*IMR	21, M.R.	M91807, L07767	
DRB1*03021[c]	DR18(3)	Dw'RSH'	–	2041, 1563	M27689	
DRB1*03022	DR18(3)	Dw'RSH'	–	GN055, GMONT	U29342, U82403	(86), M. Taylor
DRB1*0303	DR18(3)	–	–	RBL B25	M81743	
DRB1*0304	DR17(3)	–	03MIT	MIT3758	X75441	
DRB1*0305	DR17(3)	–	DR3New	U-HFI, TTO5607	L29807, U26557	S. Bowman[b]
DRB1*0306	DR3	–	–	JV1094	X90644	(87)
DRB1*0307	–	–	–	GN073	U37433	(86)
DRB1*0308	–	–	–	GN090	U47028	(86)
DRB1*0309	–	–	–	D438	X93315	(88)
DRB1*0310	–	–	–	PMR	U65585	(89)
DRB1*0311	–	–	–	UWE02	U79028	C. Hurley
DRB1*04011[c]	DR4	Dw4	–	WT51, PRIESS, MJ4, BOLETH	K02776, M17381, M20548-50, M19556	
DRB1*04012	DR4	Dw4	–	MC	X96851	(90)
DRB1*0402	DR4	Dw10	–	FS, DM24, MMCC	M15068	
DRB1*0403	DR4	Dw13	DR4 Dw13A, 13.1	SSTO, TAS	–	
DRB1*0404	DR4	Dw14	DR4 Dw14A, 14.1	BIN40, LS40, DM29	X02902, M15069, M15073, M15074	
DRB1*04051[c]	DR4	Dw15	–	KT3, JML, AHC, CRP	M15070, L13875	
DRB1*04052	DR4	Dw15	DRB1*KOM	KOM	D50889, D49952	(91)
DRB1*0406	DR4	Dw'KT2'	–	KT2	–	
DRB1*0407	DR4	Dw13	DR4 Dw13B, 13.2	JHF, R88	M37771	

HLA Alleles[a]	HLA-DR Serological Specificities	HLA-D-Associated (T-cell-defined) Specificities	Previous Equivalents	Individual or Cell Line from which the Sequence was Derived	Accession Number	References or Submitting Author(s)
DRB1*0408	DR4	Dw14	DR4-CETUS, Dw14B, 14.2	M36, RA1, SUDNA0254	M37770, L78169	B. Lo[b]
DRB1*0409	DR4	–	–	R80	M37769, M64794	
DRB1*0410	DR4	–	DR4.CB	CB, ABCC60	M81670, M36879	
DRB1*0411	DR4	–	DR4.EC	EC, HV846, HAA, JMJ	M81700, M55615, L42143, L79973	P. Stastny[b], A. Arnaiz-Villena[b]
DRB1*0412	DR4	–	AB2	ABO1078	M77672	
DRB1*0413	DR4	–	DRB1*LEV	LEV	M94460	
DRB1*0414	DR4	–	DR4 Dw10.2	VK	X65031	
DRB1*0415	DR4	–	–	NIC, HOU	X68272	
DRB1*0416	DR4	–	DR4-BELF	BEL5GB	X70788	
DRB1*0417	DR4	–	DRB1*04SAM	TOB-0070	L14481	
DRB1*0418	DR4	–	DRB1*04.N	AI7, AI8, 74DR	X71610, U38974	M. Chopek[b]
DRB1*0419	DR4	–	DR4FK	FK	L21985	
DRB1*0420	DR4	–	DRB1*04MC	AD-7863, BM29/92	L27217	
DRB1*0421	DR4	–	DR4New	SMH	X80288	
DRB1*0422	DR4	–	DR4New	D18002	U17014	
DRB1*0423	DR4	–	–	MAG	Z68503	(92)
DRB1*0424	DR4	–	DRB1*Mi	Mi	Z71541	A. Dormoy
DRB1*11011	DR11(5)	Dw5	DRw11.1	SWEIG	M11867	
DRB1*11012	DR11(5)	Dw5	–	1180, 1249	M34316	
DRB1*11013	DR11(5)	Dw5	DR11.MD, DRB1*11DCT	DR11MDA, DR11MDB, BV3402	X86803, Y07590	(93), S. Hashemi
DRB1*1102	DR11(5)	Dw'JVM'	DRw11.2	JVM	M17382	
DRB1*1103	DR11(5)	–	DRw11.3	UA-S2	M21966, M22047-49	
DRB1*11041	DR11(5)	Dw'FS'	–	FPA (FPF)[d]	–	
DRB1*11042	DR11(5)	–	–	2094	M34317	
DRB1*1105	DR11(5)	–	–	DBUG	M84188	
DRB1*1106	DR11(5)	–	DR11.CCY, 11PMH	CCY, PMH161	M98436, D14352	
DRB1*1107	b 150	–	DR11+3	BEL6KG, RMS21	X73027, X82507	
DRB1*11081	DR11(5)	–	DR11JL	JL	L21984	
DRB1*11082	DR11(5)	–	DR11HW	HW	L21983	
DRB1*1109	DR11(5)	–	DRB1*MON	BEL7MON	X75347	
DRB1*1110	b 150	–	DR11.5	BRI-6	L23986	
DRB1*1111	b 150	–	DR11.6, DR11BRA	BRI-7, 1082	L23990, L26306	
DRB1*1112	b 150	–	DR11.7	BRI-9	L23988	
DRB1*1113	DR11(5)	–	DR11-14, DR11+14	PAL-6117, 30251, EmKa, SB, BV0595, JOK	X76194, L29081, U09200, U03291, Z37162, X87677	R. Blasczyk[b]

HLA Alleles[a]	HLA-DR Serological Specificities	HLA-D-Associated (T-cell-defined) Specificities	Previous Equivalents	Individual or Cell Line from which the Sequence was Derived	Accession Number	References or Submitting Author(s)
DRB1*1114	DR11(5)	–	F1363, 115T, 94-09865	BRI-11, HN0605, DJB, BEN	U08932, Z37161, U25639, Z50187	(94)[b], A. Dormoy[b]
DRB1*1115	DR11(5)	–	DR1101v	Z.S., Z.Z., Z.Z.V., GN041, GN037	Z34824, U17380	
DRB1*1116	–	–	DRB1*OULA, DR11+13	OULA, HB7542AKG	U13009, X87200	G. Mersch[b]
DRB1*1117	–	–	UCSF-D3152, DR11-14N, 0104D0335	D3152, D3153, GN032, 950104-D0335	X77776, U17379, U33474	(95)[b]
DRB1*1118	–	–	RMS16	RMS16	X82211	
DRB1*1119	–	–	RMS117, DR11Loel	RMS117, MB, KBD	X82210, Z47353, U26558	(96)[b]
DRB1*1120	DR11(5)	–	–	CV	U25442	(97)
DRB1*1121	DR11(5)	–	–	MUL	X86976	(98)
DRB1*1122	–	–	–	ZL3096	Z49113	(99)
DRB1*1123	DR11(5)	–	DRB1*11OS	YAS	D49468	N. Nagao
DRB1*1124	–	–	7CGCE	JB, DZA95-7C	X89193, Z50746	(100), G. Fischer
DRB1*1125	DR11(5)	–	DR11x08	SimE, TAR	X91823, X97291	(101), E. Albert
DRB1*1126	DR11(5)	–	DRB.W11	WAN	X94350	W. Verduyn
DRB1*1127	DR11(5)	–	2166/1018	M.K.	X95656	(102)
DRB1*1128	–	–	–	LELIEAM	X97722	F. Guignier
DRB1*1129	–	–	DRB1*11PBT	CL1281	X99841	S. Hashemi
DRB1*1130	–	–	–	GN00153	U79027	C. Hurley
DRB1*1201	DR12(5)	Dw'DB6'	–	HERLUF, FO, HK, POPE	M27635, M27509, S48645	
DRB1*12021	DR12(5)	–	DRw12b	KI	M27510	
DRB1*12022	DR12(5)	–	DRB1*1202X	BP-9, BP-21	L34353	
DRB1*12032	DR12(5)	–	DRB1*12JBT	T00341	X83455	
DRB1*1204	–	–	MHT#12v	MHT#918	U39087	(103)
DRB1*1205	DR12(5)	–	–	JC2862	D86503	K. Tokunaga
DRB1*1301	DR13(6)	Dw18	DRw6a I	HHKB, APD	M17383, X04056	
DRB1*1302	DR13(6)	Dw19	DRw6c I	WT46, CMCC, AS	L76133	A. Arnaiz-Villena[b]
DRB1*13031[c]	DR13(6)	Dw'HAG'	–	HAG, MRS, EGS, OSC, MGA, JRS, 1181, 1183, 2708, IH, JS, MD, SK	X52451, X16649, M59798, M34320, M57599, M35182	
DRB1*13032	DR13(6)	Dw'HAG'	–	11118-CMN, 22127-EC	U41634, U34602	Y. Chen
DRB1*1304	DR13(6)	–	RB1125-14	1124, 1125	M34324	
DRB1*1305	DR13(6)	–	DRw6'PEV'	TA, JP, HS, BP, DES.DI, SUDNA0165	M57600, L78167	B. Lo[b]
DRB1*1306	DR13(6)	–	DRB1*13.MW	MW	M61899	
DRB1*1307	–	–	DRB1*JJY, DRB1*SHN	JJY, SHN	L06847, D13189	
DRB1*1308	DR13(6)	–	–	THA	L03531	

HLA Alleles[a]	HLA-DR Serological Specificities	HLA-D-Associated (T-cell-defined) Specificities	Previous Equivalents	Individual or Cell Line from which the Sequence was Derived	Accession Number	References or Submitting Author(s)
DRB1*1309	DR13(6)	–	DRB1*YUN	MJD	L23534	
DRB1*1310	DR13(6)	–	13NEW	ARA	X75442	
DRB1*1311	DR13(6)	–	1303-Like	H108, HER-2698	X74313, X75445	
DRB1*1312	–	–	DR13BRA, DR13.7	650, 651, 681, BRI-8, N170, CC75, AD-6168, DNAQC012, RMS103	L25427, L23989, D29836, L27216, X82508	
DRB1*1313[g]	–	–	–	NORH01, NORH02	U79025, U79026	C. Hurley
DRB1*1314	DR13(6)	–	1101A58, 13New	BRI-12, YAS	U08274, X82239	
DRB1*1315	–	–	83-7601	BRI-14, GN070	U08276, U32325	C. Hurley[b]
DRB1*1316	DR13(6)	–	DRB1*D86	BRI-15, JA	U08277, U25638	(104)[b]
DRB1*1317	DR13(6)	–	RB1194 13/12	RB	U03721	
DRB1*1318	DR13(6)	–	DRB1*13HZ	K27418, TH10913, ZAN FR	Z36884, X82549, Z48631	(105)[b]
DRB1*1319	DR13(6)	–	DR1308V	GN033	U17381	
DRB1*1320	DR13(6)	–	DRB1*13VHT	SR0300	Z48803	(77)
DRB1*1321	–	–	DR13TAS	ATAS	L41992	D. Maurer
DRB1*1322	–	–	–	GvdP, LI3936	X86326, X87886	M. Tilanus, F. Dufosse
DRB1*1323	–	–	–	GN079	U36827	F-M. Robbins
DRB1*1324	–	–	–	GN039	U36825	F-M. Robbins
DRB1*1325	–	–	–	MRN5981	X93924	(106)
DRB1*1326	–	–	DRB1*16WIL	WIL3966	X96396	(107)
DRB1*1327	DR13(6)	–	DRB1*13MS, DRB1*13NW	NVE 802	Z71289, U59691, X97601	(108), G. Fischer, M. Tilanus
DRB1*1328	–	–	–	DU25503	X97407	M. Varney
DRB1*1329	DR6	–	–	JC6267	D87822	K. Tokunaga
DRB1*1330	–	–	DRB1*13DAS	DAS-094	U72264	W. Greville
DRB1*1401	DR14(6)	Dw9	DRw6b I	4/w6, TEM	X04057	
DRB1*1402	DR14(6)	Dw16	–	AMALA (LIA,AZL)[d]	–	
DRB1*1403	DR1403	–	JX6	MI	–	
DRB1*1404	DR1404	–	DRB1*LY10, DRw6b.2	CEPH-137502, KGU	M34372	
DRB1*1405	DR14(6)	–	DRB1*14c	36M, 38M, SUDNA0503	M33693, M60209, L78168	B. Lo[b]
DRB1*1406	DR14(6)	–	DRB1*14.GB, 14.6	GB, SAS5041, SAS9080, SUDNA0164	M63927, M74032, L78164	B. Lo[b]
DRB1*1407	DR14(6)	–	14.7	PNG141, PNG196	M74030	
DRB1*1408	DR14(6)	–	AO1,14.8	HV178, PNG198, PNG202	M77673, M74031	
DRB1*1409	DR14(6)	–	AB4	1103	M77671	
DRB1*1410	–	–	AB3	ABCC31	M77670	
DRB1*1411	DR14(6)	–	DRw14x11	MARBrun, MARMari, MARMarg	M84238	
DRB1*1412	–	–	DRB1*YOS	YOS	D16110	
DRB1*1413	–	–	–	GRC138	L21755	

HLA Alleles[a]	HLA-DR Serological Specificities	HLA-D-Associated (T-cell-defined) Specificities	Previous Equivalents	Individual or Cell Line from which the Sequence was Derived	Accession Number	References or Submitting Author(s)
DRB1*1414	–	–	DRB1*14N	AD-2927, AD-3798, IHL AD036	L17044	
DRB1*1415	DR14(6)	–	DRB1*14af	D.M.	U02561	
DRB1*1416	–	–	DR13+14	FVA-0166	X76195	
DRB1*1417	DR14(6)	–	1412T	#15310-LN	X76938	
DRB1*1418	–	–	81-4641	BRI-13, TH6994, DR14BBD	U08275, X82552, U37264	(96)[b]
DRB1*1419	DR14(6)	–	DRB1*14MA, DRB.14a	MA-TE, AKKAL	Z38072, X86973	(98, 109)
DRB1*1420	DR14(6)	–	DRB.14o	OND-52971	X86974	(98)
DRB1*1421	–	–	DRB.14t	TGI	X86975	(98)
DRB1*1422	–	–	DRB1*BA	LS005, BA	Z50730, Z71275	(110), A. Dormoy
DRB1*1423	–	–	–	#66820	X91640	E. Albert
DRB1*1424	–	–	BY14V	BY00002	U41489	C. Hurley
DRB1*1425	–	–	HL14V	HL.BWH, MF.BWH	U41490, U41491	C. Hurley
DRB1*1426	DR14(6)	–	–	JC1980	D86502, D50865	K. Tokunaga
DRB1*1427	DR14(6)	–	–	MO52	D86504	K. Tokunaga
DRB1*1428	–	–	DRB1*14DKT	TO4138	X99839	S. Hashemi
DRB1*1429	DR14(6)	–	–	JC6094	D88310	K. Tokunaga
DRB1*0701	DR7	Dw17, Dw'DB1'	–	BURKHARDT, MANN, LBF	M16941, M17384, U09201	
DRB1*0801	DR8	Dw8.1	–	MADURA, SUDNA0140	M17386, L78166	B. Lo[b]
DRB1*08021	DR8	Dw8.2	DRw8-SPL	SPL	–	
DRB1*08022	DR8	Dw8.2	DRw8b	OLL	–	
DRB1*08031	DR8	Dw8.3	DRw8-TAB	TAB089	–	
DRB1*08032	DR8	Dw8.3	–	KT, FO, POPE	M27511	
DRB1*08041	DR8	–	RB1066-1,DR8-V 86	1066, 1127, PM	M84446, M34315	
DRB1*08042	DR8	–	–	CAY3, CAY5, CAY92, CAY96	L10402	
DRB1*0805	DR8	–	DR8-A74	MS	M84357	
DRB1*0806	DR8	–	DR8.6	RBL B24, RBL B124, SET, BOU, ALG, C.R., SUDNA0095	M87543, M86590, Z32685, L78165	B. Lo[b]
DRB1*0807	DR8	–	DR8BZ	AG, RG, L2, L4, TIC03, TIC04, TIC06	L22341, L28096	
DRB1*0808	DR8	–	08New	ETH3754	X75443	
DRB1*0809	DR8	–	DR8.7, DRB1*8.2V	BRI-10, JB44585	L23987, D45046	(111)[b]
DRB1*0810	DR8	–	LP10-1	K.R., R.R., TH10559	L19054, X82553	
DRB1*0811	DR8	–	DR8TL, DR8New	ARA016, ARAC25, JR	L29082, L32810	
DRB1*0812	DR8	–	DRB#52	4390, DRB#52	X88854, U36836	(112), M. Chopek
DRB1*0813	–	–	DRB#47	DRB#47	U36571	M. Chopek
DRB1*0814	DR8	–	DR8WE	WE, KE	U24179	(96)

HLA Alleles[a]	HLA-DR Serological Specificities	HLA-D-Associated (T-cell-defined) Specificities	Previous Equivalents	Individual or Cell Line from which the Sequence was Derived	Accession Number	References or Submitting Author(s)
DRB1*0815	–	–	DRB1*08Taree	TDS-023	U63802	(113)
DRB1*0816	–	–	DRB1*08JST	ML0273	X99840	S. Hashemi
DRB1*09012	DR9	Dw23	–	DKB, 09012, PMR, ISK	M17387, U66826, D89917	(114)[b], A. Arnaiz-Villena[b]
DRB1*1001	DR10	–	–	RAJI, NASC	M20138	
DRB3*01011[c]	DR52	Dw24	DR3 III, DRw6a III	AVL, HHKB, DM28, DM29, CMCC	X04055, X04058	
DRB3*01012	DR52	Dw24	–	PMR	U66825	(89)
DRB3*01013	DR52	Dw24	DRB3*MOBD	MO, BD	X99771	M. Guttridge
DRB3*0102	–	–	DRB3*N409	409/96-UKN	Y08063	M. Guttridge
DRB3*0201	DR52	Dw25	DRw6b III	4/w6, DM24	M17380, V00522	
DRB3*0202	DR52	Dw25	pDR5b.3	SWEIG, WT49	X99690	M. Tilanus[b]
DRB3*0203	DR52	b 150	DRB3.02p	POS	X86977	(98)
DRB3*0204	–	–	–	SCHT	X91639	E. Albert
DRB3*0205	–	–	DRB3*02-03v	GN068	U36826	F-M. Robbins
DRB3*0206	–	–	DRB3*02MT	BV1661	X95760	S. Hashemi
DRB3*0301	DR52	Dw26	–	WT46, CMCC	–	
DRB4*01[e]	DR53	–	–	LBF, DKB, BURKHARDT, KT3, PRIESS, FS, DM24, DM29, MMCC	M17385, M17388, M15071-2, K02775	
DRB4*0101101	DR53	–	–	MANN	M16942	
DRB4*0102	DR53	–	DRB4*ICML	C.M.L.	L08621	
DRB4*0103101	DR53	–	–	MJ4, BOLETH	M15178, M20555, M19556	
DRB4*0103 102N	DR'Blank'	–	DRB4 null	DBB	D89918	(114)[f]
DRB4*0104	–	–	DRB4*CR210	69-218, 76-394	X92712	(115)
DRB4*0105	DR53	–	DRB4New	17345	Y09313	(116)
DRB4*0201N	DR'Blank'	–	DRB4*VI	GN016	U50061, U70543, U70544	F-M. Robbins
DRB4*0301N	DR'Blank'	–	DRB4*v2	GN017	U70542	F-M. Robbins
DRB5*01011[c]	DR51	Dw2	DR2A Dw2	PGF, ROF-NL	M17377, M16954, M20429	
DRB5*01012	DR51	Dw2	–	GN00152	U66721	C. Hurley
DRB5*0102	DR51	Dw12	DR2A Dw12	BGE, DHO	M16955, M30182, M16086	(78)[b]
DRB5*0103	–	–	DRB5.Oli	IND-24, IND-59	X86978	(98)
DRB5*0104	–	–	DRB5*0101V	GN045	U31770	F-M Robbins
DRB5*0105	–	–	–	CP5570	X87210	(117)
DRB5*0106	–	–	DRB5*New	ZL4062	Z83201	J-M. Tiercy
DRB5*0107	–	–	DRB5*01CBT	WI01846	Y09342	S. Hashemi

HLA Alleles[a]	HLA-DR Serological Specificities	HLA-D-Associated (T-cell-defined) Specificities	Previous Equivalents	Individual or Cell Line from which the Sequence was Derived	Accession Number	References or Submitting Author(s)
DRB5*0201	DR51	Dw21	DR2A Dw21	AZH	M16956, M30181	
DRB5*0202	DR51	Dw22	DR2A Dw22	REM (RML)[d], FJO, MN-2	M20503, M15992, M32578	(78, 118)[b]
DRB5*0203	DR51	–	DRB5*HK	HK55	M91001	
DRB5*0204	–	–	–	GN00151	U59685	C. Hurley
DRB6*0101	–	–	DRBσ*0101, DRBX11	BAC, BRO-2, HOM-2, KAS116, MZ070782, HON, SAS6211	X53357, M83892	
DRB6*0201	–	–	DRBX21, DRBVI	PGF, D0208915, CGG, BA, E4181324	M77284-7, X53358, M83893	
DRB6*0202	–	–	DRBσ*0201, DRBX22, DRB6III	RML, KAS011	M83204, M83894	
DRB7*01011	–	–	DRBψ1	BOLETH, BH13	K02772-4, L31617	
DRB7*01012	–	–	–	PITOUT	L31618	

[a]Allele names given in bold type have been assigned since the 1995 Nomenclature report.
[b]This reference is to a confirmatory sequence.
[c]This sequence has been previously assigned with a four or five digit allele name.
[d]Cell line is also known by alternative name.
[e]These sequences can only be assigned a two digit allele name due to incomplete sequence information.
[f]This reference is to a corrected sequence.
[g]This sequence name has been reinstated.

TABLE 6. Designations of HLA-DQ alleles.

HLA Alleles[a]	HLA-DR Serological Specificities	HLA-D-Associated (T-cell-defined) Specificities	Previous Equivalents	Individual or Cell Line from which the Sequence was Derived	Accession Number	References or Submitting Author(s)
DQA1*0101	–	Dw1	DQA 1.1, 1.9	LG2, BML, KAS116	L34082	
DQA1*01021	–	Dw2, w21, w19	DQA 1.2, 1.19, 1.AZH	PGF, LB, CMCC, AZH, WT46, DRA, ROF-NL, EMJ	M20431, L34083	
DQA1*01022	–	Dw21	–	KAS011	L34084	
DQA1*0103	–	Dw18, w12, w8, Dw'FS'	DQA 1.3, 1.18, DRw8-DQw1	APD, TAB, FPF, WVB, 2012, E4181324	M34323, L34085	
DQA1*0104	b 150	Dw9	b 150	1183, 2013, 2012, 2708, 31227ABO, EK, KOSE, DEK, REN	M34314, L34086	
DQA1*0105	–	–	–	AK93007, 1183, 2708	L42625, L46877	(119, 120)
DQA1*0201	–	Dw7, w11	DQA 2, 3.7	LG-10, BEI, DM24, DM28, DM29, MOU	L34087	
DQA1*03011	–	Dw4, w10, w13, w14, w15	DQA 3, 3.1, 3.2	MMCC, JY, NIN, BML, DM24, DM29, BOLETH	M29613, M29616, L34088	

HLA Alleles[a]	HLA-DR Serological Specificities	HLA-D-Associated (T-cell-defined) Specificities	Previous Equivalents	Individual or Cell Line from which the Sequence was Derived	Accession Number	References or Submitting Author(s)
DQA1*0302	–	Dw23	DQA 3, 3.1, 3.2, DR9-DQw3	ISK, DKB, YT	M11124, L34089	
DQA1*0303	–	–	–	YT	L34089, L46878	(119)
DQA1*0401	–	Dw8, Dw'RSH'	DQA 4.2, 3.8	ARC, 2041, MADURA, SPL (SPACH)[c]	M33906, L34090	
DQA1*0501[d]	–	Dw3, w5, w22	DQA 4.1, 2	SWEIG	–	
DQA1*05011	–	Dw3	DQA 4.1, 2	RAJI, CMCC, VAVY	X00370, K01160, L34091	
DQA1*05012	–	Dw5	DQA 4.1, 2	MG3	–	
DQA1*05013	–	Dw22	DQA 4.1, 2	REM (RML)[c], BM16	M20506, L34092	
DQA1*0502	–	–	–	EMA	U03675	
DQA1*0503	–	Dw16	–	AMALA	L34093	
DQA1*0601	–	Dw8	DQA 4.3	LUY	L34094	
DQB1*0501	DQ5(1)	Dw1	DQB 1.1, DRw10-DQw1.1	LG2, 45.1, BML, MVL, JR, MDR, WG, DC, KAS116	X03068, M65044, L34101	
DQB1*0502	DQ5(1)	Dw21	DQB 1.2, 1.21	AZH, FJO, KAS011	L34102	
DQB1*05031	DQ5(1)	Dw9	DQB 1.3, 1.9, 1.3.1	WT52, HU129, HU128, EK	M65047, L34103, L40180	(119)[b]
DQB1*05032	DQ5(1)	Dw9	DQB 1.3, 1.9, 1.3.2	AP106, AP109, AP110, AP115	–	
DQB1*0504	DQ5(1)	–	DQB 1.9	DG, R.F.	M65046, M94773	
DQB1*06011	DQ6(1)	Dw12, w8	DQB 1.4, 1.12	AKIBA, BGE, TAB, E4181324, B.H., B.S., E4181324	L34104, X89194, L40181	(119, 121)[b]
DQB1*06012	DQ6(1)	Dw12, w8	DQB1*0601var.	Sk, Rb	M86740	
DQB1*0602	DQ6(1)	Dw2	DQB 1.5, 1.2	PGF, VYT, 2041, ROF-NL, AMAI	M20432, M65048, L34105	
DQB1*0603	DQ6(1)	Dw18, Dw'FS'	DQB 1.6, 1.18	WVB, APD, FPF, 2012, OMW	M65050, M34322, L34106	
DQB1*0604	DQ6(1)	Dw19	DQB 1.7, 1.19	CMCC, DAUDI, DM23, LD, WG, EMJ	M65051, L34107	
DQB1*06051	DQ6(1)	Dw19	DQB 1.8, DQBSLE, 1.19b, 2013-24	CI, KT, MR, 2013	M36472, M34321, M65052	
DQB1*06052	DQ6(1)	Dw19	DQB1*MDvR-1	BEN53	L26325	
DQB1*0606	–	b 150	DQB1*WA1	LINE66	M86226	
DQB1*0607	–	–	DQB1*06BRI1	08-2779-0	M87041	
DQB1*0608	–	–	DQB1*06BRI2	R.W.	M87042	
DQB1*0609	DQ6(1)	–	DQB1*06AA, DQB1New	HO301, TRACHT, N076, AK93022	L19951, L27345, D29918, L42626	S. Yasunaga[b]
DQB1*0610	–	–	DQB1MC	M.M., M.G.	X86327	(122)
DQB1*0611	DQ1	–	UNM-95-228	#MUD0130-14998	U39086	(123)
DQB1*0612	DQ1	–	DQB1*06GB	GB002	X96420	(124)
DQB1*0201	DQ2	Dw3	DQB 2	WT49, CMCC, QBL, MZ, LD, VW, MOR, JNP, DM24, DM28, DM29, BEI, VAVY	K02405, M65043, M81140, L40179	(119)[b]

HLA Alleles[a]	HLA-DR Serological Specificities	HLA-D-Associated (T-cell-defined) Specificities	Previous Equivalents	Individual or Cell Line from which the Sequence was Derived	Accession Number	References or Submitting Author(s)
DQB1*0202	DQ2	Dw7	DQB 2	BURKHARDT, BH, MOU	M81141, U07848, L34095	
DQB1*0203	DQ2	–	DQB1*02DL	RAQ, CAUCA254, CAUCA288, DL-13	Z35099, U33329, U39089, U39090	(125, 126), I. Fajardy
DQB1*0301	DQ7(3)	Dw4, w5, w8, w13	DQB 3.1	SWEIG, DQB37, NIN, JHA, JR, JME, DC, JGL, LUY, BML, DM23, MG3, AMALA	M65040, L34096	
DQB1*0302	DQ8(3)	Dw4, w10, w13, w14	DQB 3.2	BOLETH, FS, BIN40, WT51, DM24, DM29, MMCC, JS, VW, JNP, JOP	M65038, K01499, L34097	
DQB1*03032	DQ9(3)	Dw23, w11	DQB 3.3	DBB, KOZ, 5112.103, DKB	M65039, M60028, L34098	
DQB1*0304	DQ7(3)	–	DQB1*03HP, *03new	HP, RG, M.M.	M74842, M83770, X76553	
DQB1*0305	DQ8(3)	–	DQB1*03KC	G.P., M.A.	X69169, X76554	
DQB1*0306	DQ3	–	DQB1*MAT	MAT	D78569	(127)
DQB1*0307	–	–	DQB1*D4	D4	Z49215	(128)
DQB1*0401	DQ4	Dw15	DQB 4.1, Wa	KT3, YT	M13279, L34099	
DQB1*0402	DQ4	Dw8, Dw'RSH'	DQB 4.2, Wa	ARC, OLN, MZ, 2041, SPL (SPACH)[c], MADURA	M33907, M65042, L34100	

[a]Allele names given in bold type have been assigned since the 1995 Nomenclature report.
[b]This reference is to a confirmatory sequence.
[c]Cell also known by alternative name.
[d]This sequence can only be assigned a four digit allele name, as it is either published only as a protein or partial nucleotide sequence.

TABLE 7. Designations of HLA-DP alleles.

HLA Alleles[a]	HLA-D-Associated (T-cell-defined) Specificities	Previous Equivalents	Individual or Cell Line from which the Sequence was Derived	Accession Number	References or Submitting Author(s)
DPA1*0103	–	DPw4α1	BOLETH, 3.1.0, LG2, PRIESS, LB	X03100, X82390, X82392, X82389	
DPA1*0104	–	01New	SK	X78198, X81348, X82391	
DPA1*0105	DPA1*RK	DNA-RK	X96984	(129)	
DPA1*02011	–	DPA2, pDAα13B	DAUDI, AKIBA	X82394, X82393, X78199	
DPA1*02012	–	DPA1*TF	A371, L67, LB0410278	L31624, X83610	
DPA1*02021	–	2.21	CB6B	M83906, L11642, X79475, X80482, X79479	
DPA1*02022	–	2.22	LKT3, KT17, WI-L2 NS, CT46, EsSm, GIWh	M83907, L11641, X79476, X80484, X79480	
DPA1*0203	DPA1*TC48	TC48	Z48473	(130)	
DPA1*0301	–	3.1	AMAI	M83908, X79477, X81347, X79481	
DPA1*0401	–	4.1	T7526	M83909, L11643, X79478, X80483, X78200	

HLA Alleles[a]	HLA-D-Associated (T-cell-defined) Specificities	Previous Equivalents	Individual or Cell Line from which the Sequence was Derived	Accession Number	References or Submitting Author(s)
DPB1*01011	DPw1	DPB1,DPw1b	LUY, RSH, P0077, FB11	M83129, M83664, M62338, X72070	
DPB1*01012	DPw1	DPB1*WA6	LINE 101, AH1457	L19220, L27662	
DPB1*0201[c]	DPw2	DPB2.1	JY	–	
DPB1*02012	DPw2	DPB2.1	45.1, WJR076, LB	M62328, X03067, X99689	M. Tilanus[b]
DPB1*02013	DPw2	DPB2.1	CJ	X94078	(131)
DPB1*0202	DPw2	DPB2.2	QBL, DUCAF	M62329, X72071	
DPB1*0301	DPw3	DPB3	SLE, PRIESS, ETH9-0226	M62334, X02964, X03023, X78044	
DPB1*0401	DPw4	DPB4.1, DPw4a	HHKB, BOLETH, PRIESS, LC11, KAS011	M62326, M23675, K01615, N00010, M23906-9, X03022, X030025-8, X02228, X00532, X72072	
DPB1*0402	DPw4	DPB4.2, DPw4b	APD, BURKHARDT	M62327, M21886	
DPB1*0501	DPw5	DPB5	HAS, LKT3	M62333, X72073	
DPB1*0601	DPw6	DPB6	JMOS, FB11	M62335, X72074	
DPB1*0801	–	DPB8	PIAZ	M62331	
DPB1*0901	–	DPB9, DP'Cp63'	TOKUNAGA	M62341, X72075	
DPB1*1001	–	DPB10	BM21, SAVC	M85223, M62342, X72076	
DPB1*11011	–	DPB11	CRK, AVE G	M62336, X78046	
DPB1*11012	–	–	AH696	L23399	
DPB1*1301	–	DPB13	NB, KAS116	M62337, X72077	
DPB1*1401	–	DPB14	8268, KAS011	M31778, M62343, X72078	
DPB1*1501	–	DPB15	PLH	M31779, M62339, X72079	
DPB1*1601	–	DPB16	JRA, WT46	M31780, M62332, X72080	
DPB1*1701	–	DPB17	JRAB, LBUF	M31781, M62344, X72082	
DPB1*1801	–	DPB18	JCA	M62340	
DPB1*1901	–	DPB19	CB6B	M62330, X72081	
DPB1*20011	–	Oos, DPB-JA	OOS, ARENT, BEL8-CC	M58608, M63508	
DPB1*20012	–	DPB1*BRI6	NT	M97685	
DPB1*2101	–	DPB-GM, DPB30, NewD	GM, PEI52, PEI74, C1, T7527	M77659, M83915, M84621, M80300	
DPB1*2201	–	DPB1*AB1, NewH	HV152, HV385, SAS60103, SAS60106	M77674, M83919	
DPB1*2301	–	DPB32, NewB	D0208915, UK3082, UK5496, PT35, IT22, I132	M83913, M84014	
DPB1*2401	–	DPB33, NewC	UK7430	M83914	
DPB1*2501	–	DPB34, NewE	PEI46	M83916	
DPB1*26011	–	DPB31, WA2	LINE70	M86229	
DPB1*26012	–	DPB1*WA8	4-BEN NO2	L24387	
DPB1*2701	–	DPB23, WA3	LINE92, H033	M84619, M86230	
DPB1*2801	–	DPB21, JAVA2	I57, I147, JOG1489	M84617, L00599	

HLA Alleles[a]	HLA-D-Associated (T-cell-defined) Specificities	Previous Equivalents	Individual or Cell Line from which the Sequence was Derived	Accession Number	References or Submitting Author(s)
DPB1*2901	–	DPB27, NewG	RBLB66, NG105, NG113, PNG112, PNG177, SCZ244	M84625, M83918, L01467	
DPB1*3001	–	DPB28	AH1377, EB5, ETH-0245	M84620, X78045	
DPB1*3101	–	DPB22, NewF, JAVA1	I68, I147, I6, PEI03, JOG1427, JOG1471	M84618, M83917, L00598	
DPB1*3201	–	DPB24, NewI	NG78, PNG167	M84622, M85222	
DPB1*3301	–	DPB25	HO23	M84623	
DPB1*3401	–	DPB26	HO26, DH67	M84624	
DPB1*3501	–	DPB29	AH1450, AH521	M84626	
DPB1*3601	–	New A, SSK2	SASBE41, THM1, KT	M83912, D10479, D10882	
DPB1*3701	–	DPB1*WA4	LINE41	M87046	
DPB1*3801	–	SSK1	THKK	D10478	
DPB1*3901	–	DPB1*BRI4	EM, ETH-0203	M97686, X78043	
DPB1*4001	–	DPB1*BRI5, WA5	5D, LINE103, LINE105, LINE116, LINE117, LINE119, EB39, HO62	M97684, L19219, L23400	
DPB1*4101	–	DPB2.3	HT	D13174	
DPB1*4401	–	STCZ	SCZ259, SCZ244	L01466	
DPB1*4501	–	DPB1*NM	C212	L09236	
DPB1*4601	–	DPB1*NIB	V.E.C., R130	L07768, L31817	
DPB1*4701	–	DPB1*02KY, *SUT	SAJ008, SAJ119, SUT	D14344, D10834	
DPB1*4801	–	–	SE107	L17314	
DPB1*4901	–	–	HO21	L17313	
DPB1*5001	–	–	DIEDE	L17311	
DPB1*5101	–	DPB1*WA7, *EA1, *JYO	C2#3, 15-BEN, NMDP#00800-2553-8, JYO	L17310, L19219, L27073, D28809	
DPB1*5201	–	–	HO82	L22076	
DPB1*5301	–	–	EB26	L22077	
DPB1*5401	–	DPB1 New2	ETH-0222	X78042	
DPB1*5501	–	DPB1 New3, DPBGUY	ETH-0271, J.M.	X78041, X80331	
DPB1*5601	–	DPB1-R90	R90	L31816	
DPB1*5701	–	DPBMYT4220	H.R.	X80752	
DPB1*5801	–	DPB1newAW	HAM006	X82123, X85966	
DPB1*5901	–	–	GA Au, HBO1242, HBO1243, HBO1244, 0000-5922-0	Z47806, U29534, U59422	(132, 133), A. Dormoy
DPB1*6001	–	–	JN, BPN	U22313	(134)
DPB1*6101N	DP'Blank'	–	ZN	U22312	(134)
DPB1*6201	–	–	LE, CT	U22311	(134)
DPB1*6301	–	DPB1*IsOr	IsOr	U34033	(135)
DPB1*6401N	DP'Blank'	DPB1*IsAr	IsAr	U34032	(135)
DPB1*6501	–	–	E.L.	X91886	(136)
DPB1*6601	–	DPB1*BR	DNA-128	X96986	(137)
DPB1*6701	–	DPB1*TF	DNA-TF	X96985	(138)
DPB1*6801	–	DPB1*BAC	BAC1283, 902-258-3	Z70731, U59440	(133), A. Dormoy

HLA Alleles[a]	HLA-D-Associated (T-cell-defined) Specificities	Previous Equivalents	Individual or Cell Line from which the Sequence was Derived	Accession Number	References or Submitting Author(s)
DPB1*6901	–	–	SBD3497	X97406	M. Varney
DPB1*7001	–	–	900-132-2	U59441	(133)
DPB1*7101	–	–	905-967-6, I045	U59438	(133)
DPB1*7201	–	–	0014-3022-2	U59439	(133)
DPB1*7301	–	–	0076-0684-1	U59437	(133)

[a]Allele names given in bold type have been assigned since the 1995 Nomenclature report.
[b]This reference is to a confirmatory sequence.
[c]This sequence can only be assigned a four digit allele name, as it is either published only as a protein or partial nucleotide sequence.

TABLE 8. Designations of HLA-DM alleles.

HLA Alleles[a]	Previous Equivalents	Individual or Cell Line from which the Sequence was Derived	Accession Number	References
DMA*0101	RING6	JY, MANN	X62744	
DMA*0102	DMA-Ile 140	AZL	Z24753	
DMA*0103	DMA3.2	HOM-2	U04878	
DMA*0104	DMA3.4	BM21	U04877	
DMB*0101	RING7	JY, MANN	Z23139	
DMB*0102	DMB-Glu 143	YAR	Z24750	
DMB*0103	DMB-Thr 179	BM16	Z24751	
DMB*0104	DMB3.4	CEPH 23-01	U00700	
DMB*0105	HY595, DMB*KV1	HY595, H.S.K.	D32055, U16762	(139, 140)

[a]Allele names given in bold type have been assigned since the 1995 Nomenclature report.

TABLE 9. Designations of TAP alleles.

TAP Alleles	Previous Equivalents	Individual or Cell Line from which the Sequence was Derived	Accession Number
TAP1*0101	RING4, PSF(Y3), TAP1A	U937, LCL721.45, HB00028, HB00032	X57522, X57521, L21204
TAP1*02011	TAP1B	CK	L21206
TAP1*02012	TAP1E	HEH	L21205
TAP1*0301	TAP1C	JT	L21208
TAP1*0401	TAP1D	HB00031	L21207
TAP2*0101	RING11A, TAP2A	CEM-CCRF	M84748
TAP2*0102	TAP2E	JY	Z22936
TAP2*0103	TAP2F	S-2	U07844
TAP2*0201	RING11B, TAP2B	DX3	Z22935

TABLE 10. List of allele names which have been deleted.

Old name now deleted	New Name	Reason for change
A*2401	–	Sequence shown to be in error.
A*2412	A*2408	Sequence shown to be in error.
A*3005	A*3004	Sequence shown to be in error.
A*31011	A*31012	Sequence shown to be in error.
A*3302	A*3303	Sequence shown to be in error.
B*0701	–	Sequence shown to be in error.
B*27051	B*27052	Sequence shown to be in error.
B*39012	B*39011	Sequence shown to be in error.
B*4401	B*4402	Sequence shown to be in error.
B*7901	B*1518	Sequence renamed.
Cw*0101	Cw*0102	Sequence shown to be in error.
Cw*0201	Cw*02022	Sequence shown to be in error.
Cw*0301	Cw*0304	Sequence shown to be in error.
Cw*0601	Cw*0602	Sequence shown to be in error.
Cw*1101	–	Sequencing artefact.
Cw*1201	Cw*12022	Sequence shown to be in error.
Cw*1401	Cw*1402	Sequence shown to be in error.
Cw*1501	Cw*1502	Sequence shown to be in error.
Cw*1603	Cw*1403	Sequence shown to be in error.
DRB1*0702	DRB1*0701	Sequence shown to be in error.
DRB1*09011	DRB1*09012	Sequence shown to be in error.
DRB1*12031	DRB1*1201	Sequence shown to be in error.
DRB1*1313	DRB1*1313	Deleted then reinstated, see text.
DRB1*1606	DRB1*1605	Sequence shown to be in error.
DRB4*0101102N	DRB4*0103102N	Sequence shown to have been named incorrectly.
DQA1*03012	DQA1*0302	Sequence shown to be in error.
DQB1*03031	DQB1*03032	Sequence shown to be in error.
DPA1*0101	DPA1*0103	Sequence shown to be in error.
DPA1*0102	DPA1*0103	Sequence shown to be in error.
DPB1*02011	DPB1*02012	Sequence shown to be in error.
DPB1*0701	–	Named never assigned
DPB1*1201	–	Named never assigned
DPB1*4201	DPB1*3101	Sequence shown to be in error.
DPB1*4301	DPB1*2801	Sequence shown to be in error.

TABLE 11. Newly recognised and renamed serological specificities.

Previous name	New designation
AX'BG', A'Blank'	A80
B7Qui	B2708
B7801	B78
B'DT', B7x40, B7x48	B81

TABLE 12a. Complete listing of recognized serological and cellular HLA specificities.

A	B	C	D	DR	DQ	DP
A1	B5	Cw1	Dw1	DR1	DQ1	DPw1
A2	B7	Cw2	Dw2	DR103	DQ2	DPw2
A203	B703	Cw3	Dw3	DR2	DQ3	DPw3
A210	B8	Cw4	Dw4	DR3	DQ4	DPw4
A3	B12	Cw5	Dw5	DR4	DQ5(1)	DPw5
A9	B13	Cw6	Dw6	DR5	DQ6(1)	DPw6
A10	B14	Cw7	Dw7	DR6	DQ7(3)	
A11	B15	Cw8	Dw8	DR7	DQ8(3)	
A19	B16	Cw9(w3)	Dw9	DR8	DQ9(3)	
A23(9)	B17	Cw10(w3)	Dw10	DR9		
A24(9)	B18	Dw11(w7)	DR10			
A2403	B21	Dw12	DR11(5)			
A25(10)	B22	Dw13	DR12(5)			
A26(10)	B27	Dw14	DR13(6)			
A28	B2708	Dw15	DR14(6)			
A29(19)	B35	Dw16	DR1403			
A30(19)	B37	Dw17(w7)	DR1404			
A31(19)	B38(16)	Dw18(w6)	DR15(2)			
A32(19)	B39(16)	Dw19(w6)	DR16(2)			
A33(19)	B3901	Dw20	DR17(3)			
A34(10)	B3902	Dw21	DR18(3)			
A36	B40	Dw22				
A43	B4005	Dw23	DR51			
A66(10)	B41					
A68(28)	B42	Dw24	DR52			
A69(28)	B44(12)	Dw25				
A74(19)	B45(12)	Dw26	DR53			
A80	B46					
	B47					
	B48					
	B49(21)					
	B50(21)					
	B51(5)					
	B5102					
	B5103					
	B52(5)					
	B53					
	B54(22)					
	B55(22)					
	B56(22)					
	B57(17)					
	B58(17)					
	B59					
	B60(40)					
	B61(40)					
	B62(15)					
	B63(15)					
	B64(14)					
	B65(14)					

A	B	C	D	DR	DQ	DP
	B67					
	B70					
	B71(70)					
	B72(70)					
	B73					
	B75(15)					
	B76(15)					
	B77(15)					
	B78					
	B81					
	Bw4					
	Bw6					

TABLE 12b. Broad, splits and associated antigens. The listing of broad specificities in parenthesis after a narrow specificity, e.g., HLA-A23(9) is optional. The following is a list of those specificities which arose as clear-cut splits of other specificities and of associated antigens (#) which are variants of the original broad specificity and not splits as previously defined.

Original Broad Specificities	Splits and Associated Antigens#
A2	A203#, A210#
A9	A23, A24, A2403#
A10	A25, A26, A34, A66
A19	A29, A30, A31, A32, A33, A74
A28	A68, A69
B5	B51, B52, B5102#, B5103#
B7	B703#
B12	B44, B45
B14	B64, B65
B15	B62, B63, B75, B76, B77
B16	B38, B39,B3901#,B3902#
B17	B57, B58
B21	B49, B50, B4005#
B22	B54, B55, B56
B27	B2708#
B40	B60, B61
B70	B71, B72
Cw3	Cw9, Cw10
DR1	DR103#
DR2	DR15, DR16
DR3	DR17, DR18
DR5	DR11, DR12
DR6	DR13, DR14, DR1403#, DR1404#
DQ1	DQ5, DQ6
DQ3	DQ7, DQ8, DQ9
Dw6	Dw18, Dw19
Dw7	Dw11, Dw17

TABLE 12c. Bw4 and Bw6 associated specificities. The following specificities are generally agreed inclusions of HLA epitopes Bw4 and Bw6.

Bw4:	B5, B5102, B5103, B13, B17, B27, B37, B38(16), B44(12), B47, B49(21), B51(5), B52(5), B53, B57(17), B58(17), B59, B63(15), B77(15)
	and
	A9, A23(9), A24(9), A2403, A25(10), A32(19)
Bw6:	B7, B703, B8, B14, B18, B22, B2708, B35, B39(16), B3901, B3902, B40, B4005, B41, B42, B45(12), B46, B48, B50(21), B54(22), B55(22), B56(22), B60(40), B61(40), B62(15), B64(14), B65(14), B67, B70, B71(70), B72(70), B73, B75(15), B76(15), B78, B81

Nomenclature of the Fc receptors*

IUIS Subcommittee on Nomenclature[1]

Fc receptors (FcR) that are specific for particular immunoglobulin isotypes are designated by Greek letters. Subtypes of receptors are denoted by capital Roman numerals, such as:
$Fc_\gamma RI$, II and III: Fc receptors for IgG on macrophages/monocytes and lymphocytes (numerals are in the order of affinity for IgG);
$Fc_\alpha R$, $Fc_\mu R$ and $Fc_\delta R$: Fc receptors for IgA, IgM and IgD;
$Fc_\varepsilon RI$: high-affinity receptors for IgE on mast cells and basophils;
$Fc_\varepsilon RII$: low-affinity receptors for IgE on lymphocytes, macrophages, and activated eosinophils.

Species are abbreviated as follows: hu (human), mo (mouse), rt (rat), and rb (rabbit). Subunits of receptors are designated by Greek letters α, β, γ and transcripts by a, b, c, etc. Ig-BF describes the soluble molecules having affinity for immunoglobulin.

The following definition for *Fc receptors* was agreed upon: "A group of surface membrane molecules that specifically bind homologous immunoglobulin via the Fc portion, and which putatively mediate biologic functions". The preferred abbreviation for Fc receptors is FcR, those specific for a particular *immunoglobulin isotype* being designated as $Fc_\gamma R$, $Fc_\mu R$, $Fc_\alpha R$, $Fc_\delta R$ and $Fc_\varepsilon R$.

The *animal species* of the cells that express FcR are designated by abbreviations such as hu (human), mo (mouse), rt (rat) and rb (rabbit). Although Fc receptors are present on a variety of cell types, the cell type should be left unspecified in the official nomenclature of FcR. Based on immunological and molecular characteristics of the receptors, it is recommended that capital roman numerals be used to designate *subtypes*, e.g., $Fc_\gamma RI$, $Fc_\gamma RII$, $Fc_\gamma RIII$, and $Fc_\varepsilon RI$, $Fc_\varepsilon RII$. The $huFc_\gamma RI$ is a high-affinity receptor on human monocytes/macrophages with a relative molecular mass of 72 kilodaltons (M_r 72×10^3) and has affinity for monomeric IgG; $huFc_\gamma RII$ is the 40 kDa (M_r 40×10^3) molecule on monocytes, granulocytes, platelets and B cells, having affinity for IgG; and $huFc_\gamma RIII$ is the 50–70 kDa (M_r $50–70 \times 10^3$) molecule on human granulocytes and natural killer cells and has low affinity for IgG. The mouse receptor ($moFc_\gamma RI$) has high affinity for IgG_{2a}; $moFc_\gamma RII$ refers to $\gamma 1/2b$ receptors and $moFc_\gamma RIII$ is the receptor with affinity for IgG_3. High-affinity $Fc_\varepsilon R$ on mast cells/basophils are called $Fc_\varepsilon RI$ and low-affinity $Fc_\varepsilon R$ on B cells, T cells, eosinophils, and macrophages are called $Fc_\varepsilon RII$.

It is recommended that Greek letters be used for *subunits* of receptors. For example, $rtFc_\varepsilon RI$ is composed of α, β and γ chains. Different *transcripts* of a single or related gene may be signified by a, b, etc. For example, the transcripts so far identified for $Fc_\gamma RII$ could be referred to as $Fc_\gamma RII\alpha_a$, $Fc_\gamma RII\alpha_{b1}$, and $Fc_\gamma RII\alpha_{b2}$.

There are *soluble molecules* having affinity for immunoglobulin. It is proposed that they continue to be called immunoglobulin (Ig)-*binding factors* (Ig-BF) and designated as IgG-BF, IgA-BF, IgE-BF, IgM-BF and IgD-BF. Some of these molecules are fragments of FcR. Once the structure of the fragments and their structural relationship to FcR have been established, they may be referred to as *fragments* of FcR, e.g., $F(Fc_\gamma RI)$.

---

* This terminology note was drafted by a group of experts working under the auspices of the International Union of Immunological Societies (IUIS) and has been approved by the Nomenclature Committee of the IUIS. A French translation of this article appears on page 450. Requests for reprints should be sent to Dr K.F. Austen, Department of Rheumatology and Immunology, Brigham and Women's Hospital, The Seeley G. Mudd Building (Room 604), 250 Longwood Avenue, Boston, MA 02115, USA.

[1] Participating in the preparation of this document were: Dr C.L. Anderson and Dr B. Baird (USA); Dr A. Capron (France); Dr D.H. Conrad (USA); Dr G. Delespesse (Canada); Dr W. Friedman (France); Dr R.S. Geha, Dr K. Ishizaka, Dr T. Ishizaka, Dr A. Kulczycki, Jr, Dr R.G. Lynch, Dr J.R. McGhee and Dr H. Metzger (USA); Dr C. Neuport-Sautes (France); Dr D.M. Segal, Dr R.P. Siraganian, Dr J.C. Unkeless and Dr W.O. Weigle (USA); and Dr J. Yodoi (Japan).

Reprint No. **4998**

Nomenclature of Fc receptors*

IUIS/WHO Subcommittee on Nomenclature of Fc receptors[1]

An updated nomenclature for the cellular receptors of Fc fragments of immunoglobulins is presented.

Fc receptors have been defined as follows: "A group of surface membrane molecules that specifically bind immunoglobulins via the Fc portion and which mediate biological functions." The general abbreviation for Fc receptors is FcR. The Fc receptors specific for a particular immunoglobulin isotype are designated by Greek letters: FcγR for IgG, FcμR for IgM, FcαR for IgA, FcδR for IgD and FcεR for IgE. It is recommended that no subscripts or superscripts be used. Although Fc receptors are present on a variety of cell types, the cell type should be left unspecified. In general, the animal species should also be left unspecified; but if necessary, the animal species are designated by abbreviations such as hu (human), mo (mouse), rt (rat), rb (rabbit).

The nomenclature of the *subtypes* is based on the molecular and genetic characteristics of the receptors. Capital roman numerals are used to designate the subtypes. There are three FcγR (FcγRI, FcγRII and FcγRIII) and two FcεR (FcεRI and FcεRII). So far, no subtypes have been molecularly characterized for FcαR, FcμR and FcδR.

FcγRI corresponds to CD64, FcγRII to CD32, FcγRIII to CD16, FcαR to CD89, and FcεRII to CD23. It should be noted that FcεRII is a lectin-like molecule and the only Fc receptor which does not belong to the immunoglobulin superfamily.

When a particular subtype is encoded by several genes, they are designated by capital letters. The human subtypes currently characterized are designated as follows: FcγRIA, FcγRIB and FcγRIC; FcγRIIA, FcγRIIB and FcγRIIC; FcγRIIIA and FcγRIIIB. The mouse subtype is designated by reference to the human subtype. The only gene identified for mouse FcγRII is homologous to human FcγRIIB. Therefore, the mouse subtype is designated FcγRIIB. Similarly, the only gene identified for mouse FcγRIII is homologous to human FcγRIIIA. Therefore, the mouse subtype is designated FcγRIIIA. Alternative spliced *transcripts* derived from a single gene are designated by lower case letters followed by a number. For example, there are three alternative spliced products of human FcγRIIB (b1, b2, b3) and two of FcεRII (a1, a2). If a particular spliced product is secreted by cells in soluble form, this characteristic is not specified. However, if the extracellular domain of a transmembrane receptor is cleaved to generate a soluble receptor, the lower case "s" is appropriate. For example, sFcεRII and sFcγRIIIA.

Many FcRs are multisubunit receptors. It is recommended that Greek letters be used for *subunits* of receptors. The designation FcεRI or FcγRI implies the entire receptor complex. FcεRI is composed of α, β and γ subunits. An additional level of complexity has emerged because the γ subunit of FcεRI is also a subunit of FcγRI, FcγRIIIA, and the T-cell antigen receptor (TCR) in some T cells. Similarly, the β subunit of FcεRI is also a subunit of FcγRIIIA in mast cells. It is recommended to designate these subunits as FcR-γ and FcR-β respectively. The α subunit which is unique to the receptor subtype is then designated as FcεRI-α, FcγRI-α and FcγRIIIA-α. The ζ subunit of the T-cell antigen receptor is also part of FcγRIIIA in NK cells and possibly in other cells. It is recommended to designate this subunit as TCR-ζ.

The nomenclature of the other Fc receptors involved in transport of immunoglobulins will be discussed in a future revision of the nomenclature.

---

* A French translation of this article is published on page 810. Requests for reprints should be addressed to the Chairman of the IUIS Nomenclature Committee, Professor M. Kazatchkine, Hôpital Broussais, 96 rue Didot, 75014 Paris, France.

[1] Members of the Nomenclature Subcommittee: D. Conrad, M. Cooper, W.H. Fridman, J.P. Kinet (*Chairman*) and J. Ravetch.

Reprint No. **5533**

NOMENCLATURE OF COMPLEMENT *

The term " complement " is applied to a system of factors occurring in normal serum that are activated characteristically by antigen–antibody interaction and subsequently mediate a number of biologically significant consequences.

Study of the nature of complement has been concentrated to a large extent on analysis of the process of immune haemolysis,[1] and the nomenclature proposed for complement is based primarily on the haemolytic sequence. Nevertheless, it is recognized that not only may there be pathways of complement activity that diverge from the haemolytic pathway and require the participation of factors not required for immune haemolysis, but also parts of the complement system may be activated by mechanisms distinct from the sequential interactions occurring in immune haemolysis.

Complement, as it participates in immune haemolysis, comprises 9 components. It now appears established that these 9 factors are essentially similar, although not necessarily interchangeable, in the two species most studied—man and the guinea-pig—and it appears probable that this similarity extends to other mammalian species at least. For this reason it is now proposed that a uniform nomenclature be adopted for the various species that have been studied.

Several components of complement have been shown to have enzyme activity and it is to be anticipated that such activity will be described for more, and possibly for most, components. Eventually, therefore, a nomenclature may be envisaged for complement that follows the general biochemical conventions for the naming of enzymes. The notation proposed here should therefore be regarded as provisional until the necessary information becomes available.

THE COMPONENTS OF COMPLEMENT

A numerical notation is used for those complement components participating directly in the reaction of immune haemolysis. Hitherto the numbers have been preceded by the symbol C′. It is now suggested that this usage be changed and that the symbol C be used to denote complement components.

Although it would be desirable for the numerical symbols to parallel the reaction sequence—this being the procedure followed for all the more recently described components—it nevertheless appears unjustifiable to interfere with the well-established use of C1, C2 and C4 for particular components. In the order of their reaction the complement components should therefore be designated:

C1, C4, C2, C3, C5, C6, C7, C8, C9

The numbers (and letters) denoting complement components should not be subscript.

Other designations that have been used for complement components and some of their identifying properties are listed in Table 1.

First component (C1)

The first component of human complement comprises 3 distinct protein subcomponents to which the provisional names C1q, C1r and C1s have been given. C1q was previously known as the 11S component or C′0.

Although the 3 subcomponents are separate molecules, they appear to function as a unit and to occur as a macromolecular complex *in vivo*. For these reasons it is recommended that the term C1 be used wherever possible, but that, where required, the existing nomenclature be retained for the present, although in general the use of lettered suffixes or subscripts for subcomponents should be given up.

INTERMEDIATE COMPLEXES

E is used for erythrocyte, S for a single site of initiation of complement fixation, and A for antibody in conjunction with C followed by those components which have interacted. The components enumerated after EAC denote a state of reactivity, not necessarily their physical presence.

---

* This memorandum was drafted as a result of a series of informal discussions arranged by the World Health Organization on the occasion of a number of international meetings. Those who participated in its drafting are denoted by an asterisk in the list of signatories on page 938. A French version will be published in a later issue.

[1] Immune haemolysis is the process whereby fresh normal serum (from any of a number of species) lyses red blood cells (usually from the sheep) treated with antibody to them (usually prepared in the rabbit).

TABLE 1

NOMENCLATURE OF COMPLEMENT COMPONENTS

Recommended nomenclature for complement component		Previous designation	Approximate electrophoretic mobility (human C)	Approximate sedimentation coefficient (Svedberg units) (human C)
C1	C1q	11S component, C′0	γ2	11
	C1r		β	7
	C1s	C′1-esterase (after activation)	α2	4
C4		β1E globulin	β1	10
C2			β2	6
C3		C′3c, C′3a, β1C globulin	β1	10
C5		C′3b, C′3b, β1F globulin	β1	8.7
C6		C′3e, C′3α	β2	6
C7		C′3f, C′3β	β2	6
C8		C′3a, C′3c	γ1	8
C9		C′3d, C′3d	α2	5

In current usage the intermediate complex is often written with the lower-case letter " a " suffixed to components showing enzyme or other biological activity when on that complex. For example, EAC′1a, 4, 2a, 3 represents the complex produced by the reaction of the first 4 components.

It is proposed that in future the intermediate complex should be written without suffixes, e.g., EAC1423 for the complex above. Alternatively, the example may be shortened to EAC1–3.

Where the activity of components is lost from the intermediate complex, the components concerned are deleted. Thus EAC43 represents the intermediate complex resulting from the loss of C1 and C2 activity from EAC1423.

The functional cell-membrane lesion at a site of complement fixation is denoted as S*.

Where the fragments of components fixed on the intermediate complex or the activation or inactivation of a particular reactive site are to be denoted, it is recommended that this be done in a separate description according to the conventions outlined below.

COMPLEMENT COMPONENTS SHOWING ALTERED ACTIVITY

At present, the suffix " a " is used to denote the acquisition by a component or group of components of an enzymatic or other biological activity. Thus C1a denotes the activated form of C1, which has esterase activity in relation to a number of amino-acid esters and destroys C4 and C2 in solution. The C1s subcomponent from C1a (which has been called C1-esterase) is itself enzymatically active and is therefore denoted C1sa. Similarly C(42)a denotes the activity described as C3-convertase, and C(567)a the chemotactic factor derived from C5, C6 and C7.

It is proposed to substitute for the suffix " a " a bar or rule placed over the affected component. Thus $\overline{\text{C1}}$ will replace C′1a, $\overline{\text{C42}}$ will replace C(42)a and $\overline{\text{C567}}$ will replace C(567)a.

Similarly, the loss by a complement component of a defined activity has been denoted by the suffix " i ", and it is proposed that this usage be continued. However, it is highly probable that in many cases the inactivated components represent fragments produced by cleavage of the parent molecule. When sufficient information is available to designate the inactivated components as fragments (see below), this is to be preferred.

FRAGMENTS AND CHAINS

It is anticipated that growing attention will be given to the molecular structure of individual components and that a consistent nomenclature will be helpful both for the fragments produced by peptide-bond breakage and for separated polypeptide chains.

It is proposed that fragments produced during the complement-fixation reaction by peptide-bond cleavage should be denoted in the general form C*n* a, b, c . . . As examples, the fragments of C3 and C5 showing anaphylatoxin activity are designated C3a and C5a.

Where fragments are produced artificially by peptide-bond cleavage, the enzyme or other agent used may be placed after the fragment, e.g., C3a (trypsin) for the anaphylatoxin from C3 by trypsin. Where an artificial fragment is shown to be structurally identical with a fragment produced during complement fixation, the designation of the artificial treatment may be omitted.

The mechanism of the interaction of SA with the first four components, which yields the product SAC1423, could thus be written in terms of fragments and active enzymes:

$$C4+C2 \rightleftharpoons C4,2 \xrightarrow{\overline{C1}} \overline{C4,2a} \qquad C3 \xrightarrow{\overline{C4,2a}} \overline{C4,2a,3b}+C3a$$

Polypeptide chains would in an analogous way be designated α, β, chain C*n*.

COMPLEMENT FACTORS NOT DIRECTLY INVOLVED IN THE HAEMOLYTIC SEQUENCE

A number of serum factors are known to react with the intermediate complex or with the products of

TABLE 2

FACTORS[a] OTHER THAN COMPLEMENT COMPONENTS REACTING IN THE COMPLEMENT SEQUENCE

Factor	Abbreviation or synonym in use	Approximate electrophoretic mobility	Relation to complement
$\overline{C1}$ inactivator	C1 esterase inhibitor	$\alpha 2$	Inactivates $\overline{C1}$, both fixed and in free solution. Also inhibits kallikrein and PF/Dil.[b]
C3 inactivator (Conglutinogen Activatting Factor)	KAF	$\beta 1$	Reacts with fixed C3 making this reactive with conglutinin and reducing its haemolytic and immune adherence activity
C6 inactivator		$\beta 2$	Inactivates fixed C6
Conglutinin	K	$\beta 2$	Aggregates intermediate complexes containing fixed C3 which has been acted upon by KAF (C3 inactivator)
Immuno-conglutinins	IK	γ	Autoantibodies to fixed C3 and C4
Plasmin	Fibrinolysin	$\beta 1$	Acts upon C1s to activate it to C1-esteras- and upon C3 in solution to yield a chemotactic fragment
Properdin		γ	In conjunction with naturally occurring antibodies, complement components and magnesium ions, plays a part in killing certain bacteria and neutralizing certain viruses

[a] These factors should be designated in full; if abbreviations are used, however, they should be explicitly described.

[b] Miles, A. A. & Wilhelm, D. L. (1955) *Brit. J. exp. Path.*, **36**, 71-81.

complement fixation, although they play no essential role in immune haemolysis. They are enumerated in Table 2. It is not proposed that any systematic nomenclature be devised for them at the present time apart from the application, where appropriate, of the foregoing complement-component nomenclature.

GLOSSARY OF ABBREVIATIONS

E	Erythrocyte
S	Single site of complement activation
A	Antibody
C	Complement
C1, C2 . . . C9	Complement components
SAC1234 . . . *n* SAC 1–*n*	Intermediate complexes formed by the reaction of the first *n* complement components
C*n*, a, b, c . . .	Fragments of complement components produced by peptide-bond cleavage
α, β, γ . . . chain C*n*	Polypeptide chains of complement components
$C\bar{n}$	Complement component that has acquired enzymatic or other biological activity
C*n*i	Complement component that has lost a defined activity

* * *

* K. F. AUSTEN, Robert Bent Brigham Hospital, Harvard Medical School, Boston, Mass., USA
* E. L. BECKER, Walter Reed Army Institute of Research Washington, D.C., USA
C. E. BIRO, Instituto Nacional de Cardiología, Mexico City, Mexico
* T. BORSOS, National Institutes of Health, Bethesda, Md., USA
A. P. DALMASSO, Instituto de Biología y Medicina Experimental, Buenos Aires, Argentina
W. DIAS DA SILVA, Universidade de Minas Gerais, Belo Horizonte, Brazil
H. ISLIKER, Institut de Biochimie, Université de Lausanne, Lausanne, Vaud, Switzerland
P. KLEIN, Institut für Medizinische Mikrobiologie der Johannes Gutenberg-Universität, Mainz, Federal Republic of Germany
* P. J. LACHMANN, Department of Pathology, University of Cambridge, Cambridge, England
M. A. LEON, Department of Pathology Research, St Luke's Hospital, Cleveland, O., USA
* I. H. LEPOW, Health Center, University of Connecticut, Hartford, Conn., USA
* M. M. MAYER, School of Medicine, Johns Hopkins University, Baltimore, Md., USA
* H. J. MÜLLER-EBERHARD, Scripps Clinic and Research Foundation, La Jolla, Calif., USA
* R. A. NELSON, University of California, San Diego, Calif., USA
U. NILSSON, Institute of Medical Microbiology, Lund, Sweden (present address: Hospital of the University of Pennsylvania, Philadelphia, Pa., USA)
I. NISHIOKA, National Cancer Research Institute, Tokyo, Japan
* H. J. RAPP, National Institutes of Health, Bethesda, Md., USA
* F. S. ROSEN, Children's Hospital, Harvard Medical School, Boston, Mass., USA
* Z. TRNKA, Immunology, World Health Organization, Geneva, Switzerland
P. A. WARD, Armed Forces Institute of Pathology, Washington, D.C., USA
A. C. WARDLAW, School of Hygiene, University of Toronto, Toronto, Canada

Nomenclature of the alternative activating pathway of complement*

This terminology note outlines for the first time a standard nomenclature for the alternative activating pathway of complement. It was drafted by a group of experts working under the auspices of the International Union of Immunological Societies (IUIS), and has been approved by the Nomenclature Committee of the IUIS.

The complement system, as it is now understood, is comprised of two pathways for activation, the classical and alternative activating pathways, and a single membrane attack pathway which is common to both activating pathways. A previous document (*1*) outlined a standard nomenclature for the third complement component, C3, and for the components of both the classical activating pathway, C1, C4, and C2, and the membrane attack pathway, C5, C6, C7, C8, and C9. There is now sufficient agreement concerning the proteins of the alternative activating pathway of the two species studied most, man and guinea-pig, to allow the adoption of a standard nomenclature for this system.

Five proteins of the alternative pathway are designated by capital letters B, D, P, H, and I, whereas C3 retains its numerical notation. This nomenclature facilitates the writing of protein–protein complexes and cleavage fragments, and does not specify a sequentially proceeding reaction, a connotation which would be inappropriate with this pathway whose constituent proteins act in concert. Fragments of proteins that are produced during alternative activating pathway reactions are denoted by lower case letters, the lesser fragment represented by "a" and the larger fragment by "b", as in Ba and Bb. Complexes between proteins are represented by enumerating the proteins with an intervening comma, as in C3b,Bb. The loss of a defined activity by a protein, when not associated with an alteration in the primary polypeptide structure, is denoted by the letter "i" following the protein, as in Bbi, i.e., the form of Bb which has dissociated from C3b and is no longer a peptide hydrolase for C3 or C5. When a protein loses a defined activity as a consequence of peptide hydrolysis unaccompanied by fragmentation, it shall be preceded by "i", as in iC3b, i.e., the form of C3b whose α polypeptide has been hydrolysed by I in the presence of H and is not capable of forming a C3 convertase. If inactivation of a protein is accompanied by fragmentation, the "i" is not necessary as the new fragments can be described by new lower case letters. Superscripts and overbars are not recommended, as these notations are not compatible with computer terminology. These conventions are summarized in Table 1, which lists the recommended nomenclature, previous designations, and descriptions of alternative activating pathway proteins and some of the protein-protein complexes.

* This terminology note was drafted by a subcommittee of the IUIS/WHO Nomenclature Committee. The names of the members of the subcommittee are given on page 491. A French version of this article will be published in a later issue of the *Bulletin*.

Table 1. Nomenclature of the alternative activating pathway components and intermediates

Component	Former designation	Reaction products	Description
C3	Factor A	C3a	A peptide of relative molecular mass (RMM) 9000 that is hydrolysed from C3 by a C3 convertase and that possesses anaphylatoxin activity
		C3b	A major fragment, of RMM 180 000, that is derived from C3 by the hydrolytic action of a C3 convertase and that, whether bound to a particle or unbound, may participate in formation of the amplification C3 convertase
		iC3b	C3b that has been inactivated by the peptide hydrolytic action of I in the presence of H without overt fragmentation and that cannot participate in formation of the amplification C3 convertase
B	Heat labile factor; C3 proactivator; glycine-rich β-glycoprotein	Ba	An activation peptide of RMM 30 000 that is hydrolysed from B by D
		Bb	A major fragment of RMM 63 000 that is derived from B by the hydrolytic action of D and that bears a peptide hydrolase enzymatic site active on C3 and C5
		Bbi	Inactive Bb that has dissociated from C3b and that cannot hydrolyse a peptide bond in C3 and C5
D	GBGase; C3 proactivator convertase		A glycoprotein of RMM 25 000 that is a serine proteinase which hydrolyses an Arg–Lys bond in B that is complexed to C3b
P	Properdin		A glycoprotein of RMM 220 000 that can bind to C3, C3b, and C3b,Bb and that can retard dissociation of Bb from C3b
H	β1H; C3bINA-accelerator		A glycoprotein of RMM 150 000 that can bind to C3b and that can impair binding of B to C3b, accelerate dissociation of Bb from C3b, and facilitate conversion of C3b to iC3b by I
I	C3b inactivator; C4b inactivator; KAF		A glycoprotein of RMM 93 000 that is a peptide hydrolase which converts C3b to iC3b by cleavage of a bond in the α-chain
C3b,B			Magnesium-dependent reversible complex in which B may be hydrolysed to its Bb and Ba fragments by D
C3b,Bb			Amplification C3 convertase in which Bb can hydrolyse the Arg77–Ser78 bond of the α-chain of C3
C3b,Bb,C3b			Amplification C5 convertase in which Bb can hydrolyse the Arg74–x75 bond of the α-chain of C5
C3b,Bb,P C3b,Bb,C3b,P			P-stabilized amplification C3 and C5 convertases

Members of subcommittee

C. A. Alper, Center for Blood Research, Boston, MA, USA

K. F. Austen, Harvard Medical School, Brigham and Women's Hospital, Boston, MA, USA (*Chairman*)

N. R. Cooper, Scripps Clinic and Research Foundation, La Jolla, CA, USA

D. T. Fearon, Harvard Medical School, Brigham and Women's Hospital, Boston, MA, USA

I. Gigli, New York University School of Medicine, New York, NY, USA

U. Hadding, Institute of Medical Microbiology, Johannes Gutenberg University, Mainz, Federal Republic of Germany

P. J. Lachmann, Medical Research Council, Cambridge, England

P. H. Lambert, Immunology Research and Training Centre, World Health Organization, Geneva, Switzerland

I. H. Lepow, Sterling-Winthrop Research Institute, Rensselaer, New York, USA

M. M. Mayer, The Johns Hopkins University School of Medicine, Baltimore, MD, USA

H. J. Müller-Eberhard, Scripps Clinic and Research Foundation, La Jolla, CA, USA

K. Nishioka, Tokyo Metropolitan Institute of Medical Science, Tokyo, Japan

K. Pondman, Central Laboratory of the Blood Transfusion Service of the Netherlands Red Cross, Amsterdam, The Netherlands

F. S. Rosen, Harvard Medical School, Children's Hospital Medical Center, Boston, MA, USA

R. M. Stroud, Dallas, TX, USA

REFERENCES

1. Nomenclature of complement. *Bulletin of the World Health Organization*, **39**: 935-938 (1968).

Nomenclature for human complement component C2*

WHO–IUIS Nomenclature Sub-Committee[1]

This note describes the designations for variants of the human complement component C2, which were approved by the Nomenclature Committee of the International Union of Immunological Societies (IUIS).

C2 variants

The reference typing recommended by the Sixth Complement Genetics Workshop permits nine electrophoretic variants of C2 to be distinguished (Fig. 1). In addition to the common form C2 C, four acidic variants and four basic variants are observed (Table 1).

Differences in pI between variants are difficult to establish. We therefore propose to designate the variants according to their relative IEF migration, taking the distance between the two major bands of the common C2 C as a reference unit. This distance has been estimated to be approximately 0.1 pH interval (*3*). As initially proposed, the common C2 allele is called C2*C; the acidic and basic alleles are designated C2*A and C2*B, respectively (*1, 2*). The numeric symbols, corresponding to the relative migration value, clearly permit the rare acidic and rare basic variants to be differentiated. However, the most common basic variant (approximate gene frequency, 0.02 to 0.04), designated in this nomenclature as B03, may still in common usage be named C2 B. The nomenclature of all the variants tested for the Workshop is given in Fig. 1 and conforms to the guidelines of the international system for human gene nomenclature (*6*). The previously described C2 A1 and C2 A2 variants (*4, 5*) were not available for comparison. Consequently, the present note probably does not include all of the variants of C2 thus disclosed. Other variants and new variants may easily be included in this nomenclature after comparison with the currently reported variants.

References

1. **Alper, C.** Inherited structural polymorphism in human C2: evidence for genetic linkage between C2 and BF. *J. exp. med.*, **144**: 1111–1115 (1976).
2. **Jahn, I. et al.** C2 reference typing report. *Complement inflamm.*, **7**: 175–182 (1990).
3. **Meo, T. et al.** Mapping of the HLA locus controlling C2 structural variants and linkage disequilibrium between alleles $C2^2$ and Bw 15. *Eur. j. immunol.*, **6**: 916–919 (1976).
4. **Pariser, K. et al.** Evidence for silent or null gene in hereditary C2 deficiency. *J. immunol.*, **121**: 2580–2581 (1978).
5. **Raum, D. et al.** Mapping of the structural gene for the second component of complement with respect to the human major histocompatibility complex. *Am. j. hum. genet.*, **31**: 35–41 (1979).
6. **Shows, T.B. et al.** International system for human gene nomenclature. *Cytogenet. cell genet.*, **25**: 96–116 (1979).

---

* This article was drafted by a group of experts at the time of the VIth Complement Genetics Workshop (Mainz, Germany, 1989) and has been approved by the Nomenclature Committee of IUIS. A French translation appears on pages 529–530. Requests for reprints and all correspondence should be addressed to the Chairman of the IUIS Nomenclature Committee, Dr M.D. Kazatchkine, Unité d'Immunopathologie, Hôpital Broussais, 96 rue Didot, 75014-Paris, France.

[1] Members of the group of experts: G. Hauptmann (France) (*Chairman*), M. Abbal (France), C.A. Alper (USA), D. Arnold (France), F. Christiansen (Australia), R.L. Dawkins (Australia), G. Doxiadis (Germany), G. Geserick (Germany), C.M. Giles (United Kingdom), M. Hobart (United Kingdom), I. Jahn (France), M.L. Lokki (Finland), G. Mauff (Germany), S. Nakamura (Japan), G.J. O'Neill (USA), Ch. Rittner (Germany), P.M. Schneider (Germany), O.G. Segurado (Spain), I. Siemens (Germany), K. Suzuki (Japan), K. Tokunaga (Japan), and B. Uring-Lambert (France).

Reprint No. **5310**

Table 1: **The conclusive identification of C2 allotypes**[a]

New designation Old designation	A08 –	A04 AX	A03 –	A02 AT	C C	B03 B	B07 –	B08 BH	B1 BJ
Native C2	±	+	+	+	+	+	±	±	–
C2a fragment	–	–	–	–	–	+	±	±	–
Desialized C2	+	–	–	–	–	–	±	±	+
Native C2 and desialized C2	+	+	+	+	+	+	+	+	+

[a] + : method sufficient by itself for the identification of the variant.
± : results need confirmation by data obtained from other methods.
– : method not sufficient by itself for identifying the variant. Study of native and desialized C2 is necessary to identify all C2 variants.

Fig. 1. **Schematic representation of the C2 allotypes of C2 (IEF and immunoblotting of the native protein) and nomenclature of C2 variants.** The two major bands of the common form C2 C are indicated by arrows. The distance between the arrows is used as a reference unit for the estimation of the relative IEF migration distances, permitting a numeric designation. The new variant designation is indicated in bold characters.

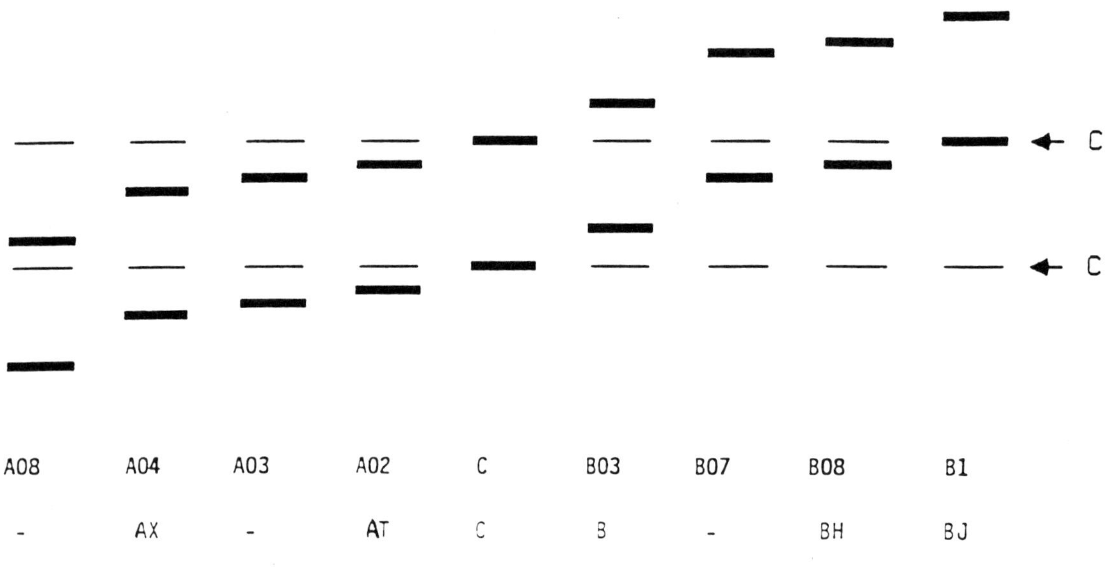

Revised nomenclature for human complement component C4*

WHO–IUIS Nomenclature Sub-Committee[1]

This note describes the recommended designations for allotypes of human complement component C4, which were approved by the Nomenclature Committee of the International Union of Immunological Societies (IUIS).

C4 nomenclature and C4 typing

General guidelines

Two polymorphic species of C4 protein with different antigenicity, designated C4A and C4B, are present in the plasma of most individuals (*2, 3*). C4A and C4B are encoded at two separate but closely linked loci within the major histocompatibility complex on the short arm of chromosome 6 (*4*). Duplications and deletion or non-expression are common for both loci. Some individuals carry hybrid C4 genes which are believed to code for aberrant proteins, some of which exhibit reversed antigenicity.

A common designation for C4 allotypes was first proposed in 1983 (*1*). The subsequent identification of aberrant proteins, the recognition of duplicated C4 genes as part of defined haplotypes with other MHC genes, and the increasing number of newly reported variants called for a revision of the nomenclature. The present revised nomenclature follows the guidelines for human gene nomenclature (*5*) and the general rules of the 1983 nomenclature statement. Since no exception has been found to the observation that the C4B protein is associated with the Chido 4 epitope and high haemolytic activity, it is recommended that the assessment of the relative haemolytic activity in an overlay on agarose gel electrophoresis containing sheep erythrocytes and C4-deficient guinea-pig serum, is used to distinguish between C4A and C4B proteins. C4B exhibits an approximately four times greater haemolytic activity than C4A (*6*). Thus, the basic typing procedure consists of immunofixation with anti-C4 antisera of proteins separated by agarose gel electrophoresis and of simultaneous haemolytic overlay as described in Table 1 of the 1983 nomenclature statement, with the exception that, in addition to neuraminidase, treatment of the samples with carboxipeptidase B (CARB-B) (*7*) should be used if the number of expressed alleles and their relative distance of migration are to be determined. Additional techniques may be necessary to identify subtype allotypes and haplotypes, including Western blotting with polyclonal or monoclonal antibodies following prolonged agarose gel electrophoresis, Rogers/Chido typing, typing of C4 alpha and beta chains, and DNA Taq1 RFLP for the recognition of gene size and duplications.

Designations of C4 allotypes

The allotypes are to be designated according to their relative electrophoretic mobility by increasing arabic numbers from the cathode to the anode for both proteins (Fig. 1 and 2, Table 1). The designation of allotypes with migration positions that are cathodal of A 1 or B 1 should be preceded by the number 9 (e.g., A 91, A 92, B 91, B 92). The two most common allotypes in all ethnic groups, A 3 and B 1, as well as the majority of the less common variants of C4, will keep their single digit numeric designation, with the exception of C4B 5, C4B 6, and C4B 7. A new designation of this region was considered to be necessary since the most common variant "B 6", which is almost invariably associated with C4A 4, HLA-B55 and DR1 or 6, has repeatedly been published as C4B 5. Thus, to avoid any further misunder-

* This article was drafted by a group of experts at the time of the VIth Complement Genetics Workshop (Mainz, Germany, 1989) and has been approved by the Nomenclature Committee of IUIS. A French translation appears on pages 536–540.

Requests for reprints and all correspondence should be addressed to the Chairman of the IUIS Nomenclature Committee, Dr M. Kazatchkine, Unité d'Immunopathologie, Hôpital Broussais, 96 rue Didot, 75014-Paris, France.

[1] Members of the group of experts: G. Mauff (Germany) (*Chairman*), M. Abbal (France), C.A. Alper (USA), F. Christiansen (Australia), M. Cuccia (Italy), R. Dawkins (Australia), G. Doxiadis (Germany), E. du Toit (South Africa), C. Giles (United Kingdom), G. Geserick (Germany), G. Hauptmann (France), M. Hobart (United Kingdom), M. Lokki (Finland), R. McLean (USA), S. Nakamura (Japan), G. O'Neill (USA), J. Partanen (Finland), Ch. Rittner (Germany), P.M. Schneider (Germany), O. Segurado (Spain), I. Siemens (Germany), K. Suzuki (Japan) and I.T. de Messias (Brazil).

Reprint No. **5311**

Fig. 1. **C4 allotypes**. Prolonged immunofixation agarose-gel electrophoresis (CARB-B and neuraminidase (NANA'se) treatment) of standard and rare allotypes submitted to the VIth Complement Genetics Workshop Reference Typing. In italics: classified allotype.

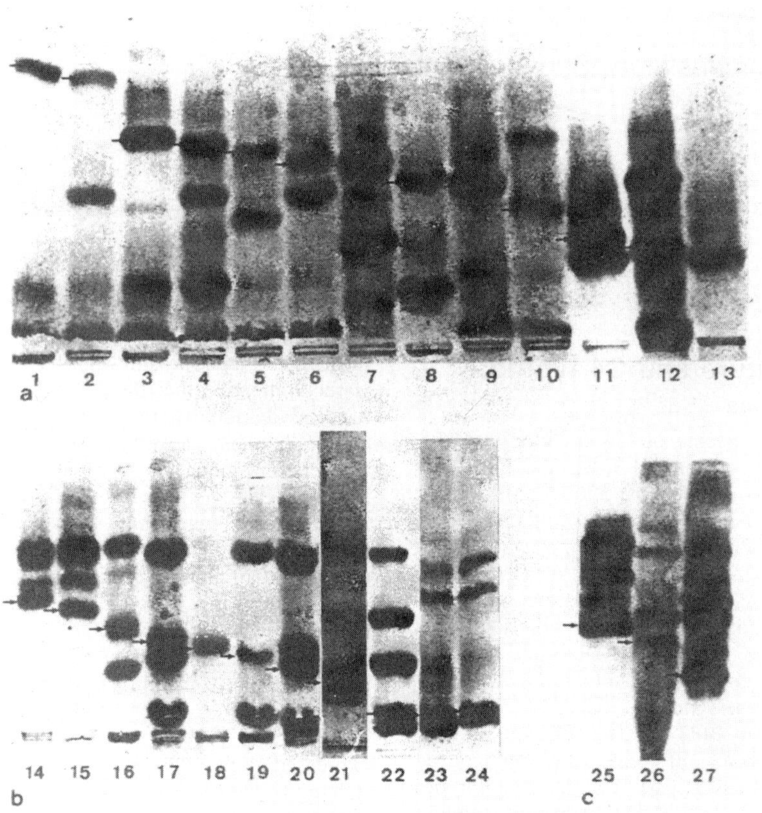

Phenotype:	C4A	B		C4A	B
a 1: WOO 001/1	*8*	1	2: CUC 001/1	*7*, 3	1
3: RIT AB	*6*	1	4: TAB 001/2	*58*, 3	3, 1
5: MAU 006/5	*55*, 2	1	6: ALP 001	*5*, 3	1
7: DUT 002/2	*45*, 12	(92)	8: MAU 037/1	*4*	2
9: MAU 015/1	*3*	1	10: MAU 006/5	55, *2*	1
11: ALP 004	*12*, 91	Q0	12: ALP 006	3, *1*	1
13: ALP 007/2	*91*	Q0			
b 14: RIT HDW	4, 3, 2	*6*	15: RIT KHH	4, 3, 2	*5*
16: TOK CWT2	4	*45*, 2	17: DOX 001/1	3	*35*, 22, 1
18: ALP 007/1	91[a]	*35*[a]	19: DAW Rob	3	*3*, 1
20: DOX 001/1	3	35, *22*, 1	21: MAU 037/1	4	*2*
22: MAU 006/4	4	5,3,*13*,1	23: HAU 002/2	3, 2	*12*, 1
24: TAB 001/7	3, 2	*11*, 1			
c 25: DUT 002/2	45,12	*92*	26: PAR 001/1	6, 3	1, *94*
27: TOK CWT6	4	2, 1, *96*			
(standard separation conditions)					

[a] A 91 B 35 in sample 18 could not electrophoretically be separated but were distinguished by lysis and segregation analysis.

Fig. 2. **Relative migration distances of C4 allotypes.** (VIth Complement Genetics Workshop Reference Typing)

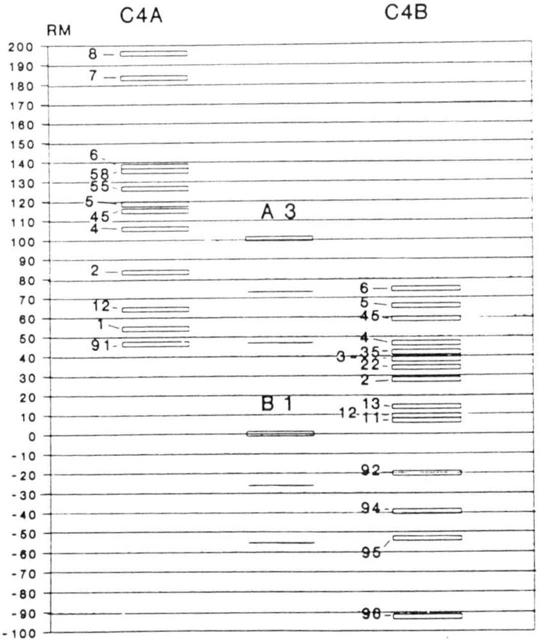

standing, the variant designated B 5 in the 1983 nomenclature will now be designated B 45; B 6 will be designated B 5, and B 7 will be designated B6. The deleted or non-expressed C4A will be designated C4A Q0; the deleted or non-expressed C4B will be designated C4B Q0.

As proposed in the earlier nomenclature, allotypes characterized by an intermediate migration between previously described allotypes will receive a two (or three) digit designation. Newly discovered allotypes should not interfere with already described variants; they should receive a one-digit-designation if they migrate outside the range of the known variants, two or three digits if they migrate between known allotypes. The classification of an allotype based on its migration may be estimated relatively to the major or minor bands observed following neuraminidase treatment of C4. A more reliable classification will result from the measurements of relative migration distances following treatment with CARB-B (the distance between C4B 1 and C4A 3 is given a reference value of 100) (Table 1) and electrophoretic side-by-side comparison.

The C4A 51, 14, 13, 11, C4B 51, 31, 29, 21, 91, 95 variants described in the 1983 nomenclature statement have not been submitted to the reference typing of the VIth Complement Genetics Workshop. C4B 31 is now considered to be identical to C4A 91 and B 29 identical to B 3. Other variants may have received new designations (e.g., C4A 51, A 91, B 51 or B 4) or belong to not yet recognized heterogeneous groups (e.g., A 14, A 13, 11, or B 21). Classification of these variants will have to wait for future reference typing.

Duplicated loci, designated as haplotype or genotype will be expressed by repeating the locus symbol: e.g., *C4A*3 A*2*; if designated as phenotype or allotype, they will be expressed in parentheses without repetition of the locus symbol: e.g., C4A (3,2).

Aberrant allotypes discovered by additional methods, e.g., Rodgers and Chido typing, Western blot with monoclonal antibodies, C4-chain typing or gene size of restriction fragment length polymorphisms (RFLPs) will not receive a special nomenclature. Subtypes should be designated by a special suffix to the main allotype.

For RFLPs, designations should indicate the probe, restriction sites (enzymes), size of the detectable fragments, and possibly their relative intensities.

C4 reference variants

A small number of standard reference variants will be available on request. They are exclusively intended for the classification of internal laboratory standards.

Addendum

Since the VIth Complement Genetics Workshop a further C4 reference typing took place during the XI International Histocompatibility Workshop in Yokohama, Japan, 1991, Ten additional C4 variants were newly discovered and characterized (see Table 2 (*10*).

References

1. **Mauff, G. et al.** Statement on the nomenclature of human C4 allotypes. *Immunobiol.*, **164**: 184–191 (1983).
2. **Awdeh, Z.L. et al.** Inherited structural polymorphism of the fourth component of human complement. *Proc. Natl Acad. Sci.*, **77**: 3576–3580 (1980).
3. **Tilley, C.A. et al.** Localization of Chido and Rodgers determinants to the C4d fragment of human C4. *Nature*, **276**: 714–716 (1978).
4. **O'Neill, G.J. et al.** Two HLA-linked loci controlling the fourth component of human complement. *Proc.*

Table 1: **Alleles of C4**[a]

Allele designation					
New	Previous	Mean RM	N	Lysis type	MAB
A Q0	A Q0	Silent allele			
A 8	A 7	197.2	1	A	nd
A 7	A 7	183.9	1	A	A
A 6	A 6	138.2 (136.3, 139.4)[b]	4	A	A
A 58	A 6	136.0	1	A	A
A 55	A 6	127.8 (127.5, 128.0)	2	A	A
A 5	A 5	119.4 (116.1, 121.1)	4	A	A
A 45	A 5	116.9	1	A	A
A 4	A 4/35	107.9	1	A	A
A 3	A 3	98.9	1	A	A
A 2	A 2	82.6	1	A	A
A 12	A 12/A 1	64.0 (59.6, 67.8)	6	A	A/B
A 1	A 1	54.2 (53.6, 54.8)	3	A	A/B
A 91	A 91/A 90/A 1/B 31	47.8 (45.3, 49.8)	6	A	B
B Q0	B Q0	Silent allele			
B 6	B 6/B 7	72.6 (72.2, 73.0)	2	B	B/A
B 5	B 5/B 6	67.3 (62.5, 70.4)	8	B	A/B
B 45	B 5	59.2	1	B	A
B 4	B 4	46.6 (46.3, 47.2)	3	B	A/B
B 35	B 3	43.5 (42.6, 44.3)	2	B	B
B 3	B 29/3/4	39.2 (37.0, 42.5)	9	B	A/B
B 22	B 22	33.2	1	B	B
B 2	B 2	29.4 (27.6, 31.2)	2	B	B
B 13	B 12	12.9 (12.7, 13.2)	3	B	A
B 12	B 12	9.5 (8.7, 10.0)	3	B	A
B 11	B 12/A 95	7.7	1	B	A
B 1	B 1	0.0	1	B	B
B 92	B 92	−20.7 (−19.7, −21.1)	2	B	B
B 94	B 94	(−40.7)[c]	1	B	B
B 95	B 95	nd	1	B	nd
B 96	B 9	(−92.6)[c]	1	B	B

[a] Abbreviations: nd, not determined. RM, relative migration value (mean value if several samples were tested; three to ten determinations per individual sample). N, number of tested samples. MAB, monoclonal antibody reactivity anti-C4A/Rg1, 2, anti-C4B/Ch1 (*8,9*).
[b] Figures in parentheses are the ranges of RM values (lowest and highest individual allotype value).
[c] Only estimates.

Table 2: **Newly discovered C4 alleles at the XI Histocompatibility Workshop, 1991**

Allele designation	Mean RM[a]	Lysis type	MAB[a]
A 62	145.9	A	A
A 3 "hybrid"	100.0	A	A+B [b]
A 22	84.6	A	A
	(83.0, 86.2) [c]		
A 19	81.2	A	A
A 95	0.0	A	B [b]
B 7	81.9	B	B
B 18	25.5	B	B
	(24.4, 26.5) [c]		
B 17	23.5	B	B
B 16	22.6	B	B
B 15	18.2	B	B

[a] RM, relative migration value (mean value if several samples were tested; three to ten determinations per individual sample); MAB, monoclonal antibody reactivity with anti-C4A/Rg1,2, anti-C4B/Ch1.
[b] Aberrant allotypes are underlined.
[c] Figures in parentheses are the ranges of RM values (lowest and highest individual allotype value).

Natl Acad. Sci., **75**: 5165–5169 (1978).

5. **Shows, T.B. et al.** Guidelines for human gene nomenclature. An international system for human gene nomenclature. *Cytogenet. cell genet.*, **46**: 11–28 (1987).
6. **Isenman, D.E. & Young J.R.** Comparison of functional properties of the human C4 isotypes. The molecular basis for the difference in immune hemolysis activity of the Chido and Rodgers isotypes of fourth human complement component. *J. immunol.*, **132**: 3019–3027 (1984).
7. **Sim, E. & Cross, S.J.** Phenotyping of human complement C4, a class-III HLA antigen. *Biochem. j.*, **239**: 763–767 (1986).
8. **Doxiadis, G. & Grosse-Wilde, H.** C4 allotyping by prolonged gel electrophoresis and immunoblotting using monoclonal and polyclonal antibodies. *Complement inflamm.*, **7**: 267–276 (1990).
9. **Giles, C.** C4: Rogers and Chido typing. *Complement inflamm.*, **7**: 213–217 (1990).
10. **Mauff, G. et al.** C4 reference typing report of the XI International Histocompatibility Workshop. *In*: Tsuji, K. et al., ed. *Histocompatibility, 1991*. Vol. 1. Oxford, Oxford University Press (in press).

Nomenclature for human complement factor B*

WHO–IUIS Nomenclature Sub-Committee[1]

In this note is recommended a unified nomenclature for allotypes and variants of human complement factor B, which was approved by the Nomenclature Committee of the International Union of Immunological Societies (IUIS).

Allotypes and subtypes

Major ("standard") BF allotypes and variants

Agarose gel electrophoresis (AGE) was originally used to describe three common allotypes and two variants of complement factor B (BF), which were named according to their electrophoretic mobility as F (fast), S (slow), F1, and "S1" (now S07) (*1, 2*): these designations are still valid. Further rare variants were found by AGE and a nomenclature analogous to that used for the C3 system was chosen for their designation (*3*).

During the VIth Complement Genetics Workshop, it was agreed that the modified alphanumeric nomenclature of factor B allotypes, according to Mauff et al. (*3*), has general acceptance and should be used in the future. The nomenclature will be applied to all BF allotypes distinguishable by standard AGE. The common alleles will be designated *BF*F* and *BF*S*. Other variants will be designated according to their relative electrophoretic mobility, using AGE, by comparison with the migration distance between the S and F1 bands, which is arbitrarily given a value of 1.0. There is the possibility for expansion with newly described variants.

The major BF allotypes and their population distribution have been reviewed (*4*). Among the six variants submitted to the VIth Complement Genetics Workshop (Reference Typing) were two new allotypes, BF F02 QL (QL = quantitatively low) and S04. A further variant, which could not be characterized by its relative electrophoretic migration with sufficient reliability, is classified as "S02". A list of the currently reported major factor B allotypes is presented in Table 1.

BF subtypes and "subtype variants"

Common subtypes of BF F. The gene product of BF*F may be split into two subtypes by IEF (isoelectric focusing) in polyacrylamide gel (*5, 6*) and agarose gel (*7*). The BF F subtypes, as well as other described rare variants, are not detectable by standard AGE. Different designations have previously been used for these variants and the standard nomenclature according to Mauff et al. (*3*) has therefore to be extended.

For practical purposes an alphabetical designation with capital letters will now be used, which is adaptable to the nomenclature of the standard allotypes. The following nomenclature should be used: FA (for the stronger *a*nodal = *a*cidic minor band) and FB (for the stronger *b*asic minor band) (Fig. 1).

Table 1: **Currently recognized variants of major ("standard") allotypes of factor B**

BF F	BF S	Non-classified	Hypomorphic
155	025	"F135"	F02QL
13	03	"F1.29"	FQL
12	035	"S02"	
115	04		
11	045		
1	05		
085	07 (formerly S1)		
08	11		
075			
065			
055			
035			
02			

* This article was drafted by a group of experts at the time of the VIth Complement Genetics Workshop (Mainz, Germany, 1989) and has been approved by the Nomenclature Committee of IUIS. A French translation appears on pages 544–546. Requests for reprints and all correspondence should be addressed to the Chairman of the IUIS Nomenclature Committee, Dr M. D. Kazatchkine, Unité d'Immunopathologie, Hôpital Broussais, 96 rue Didot, 75014-Paris, France.

[1] Members of the group of experts: G. Geserick (Germany) (*Chairman*), M. Abbal (France), C.A. Alper (USA), J. Bertrams (Germany), E. du Toit (South Africa), G. Hauptmann (France), M.L. Lokki (Finland), G. Mauff (Germany), S. Nakamura (Japan), O.G. Segurado (Spain), I. Siemens (Germany), K. Suzuki (Japan), and S. Weidinger (Germany).

Reprint No. **5312**

Fig. 1a: **BF major phenotypes and BF F subtypes as assessed by the analysis of the Ba fragment following inulin conversion of serum, immunofixation and agarose-gel isoelectric focusing (anode at top).** Some of the rare major allotypes are not detectable in the Ba fragment (e.g. BF*F1) or show unusual additional bands (BF*F055). (From ref. *16*)

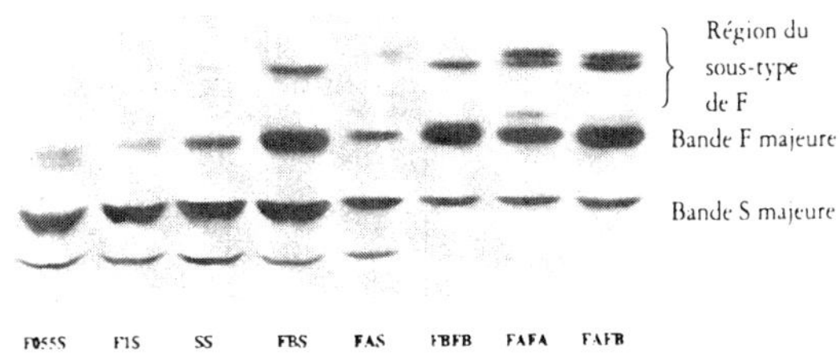

Fig. 1b: **BF major phenotypes and BF F subtypes in the Ba fragment; schematic banding pattern on agarose-gel isoelectric focusing (anode at top).** (From ref. *16*)

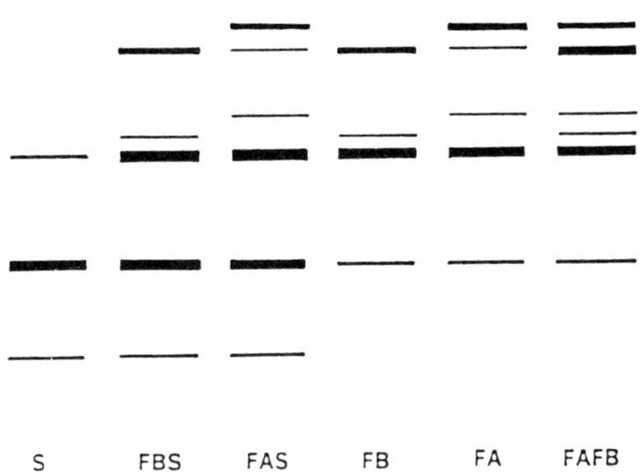

Fig. 2. **BF S variant "subtypes" in the Bb fragment following inulin conversion, immunofixation and agarose-gel isoelectric focusing (anode at top).**

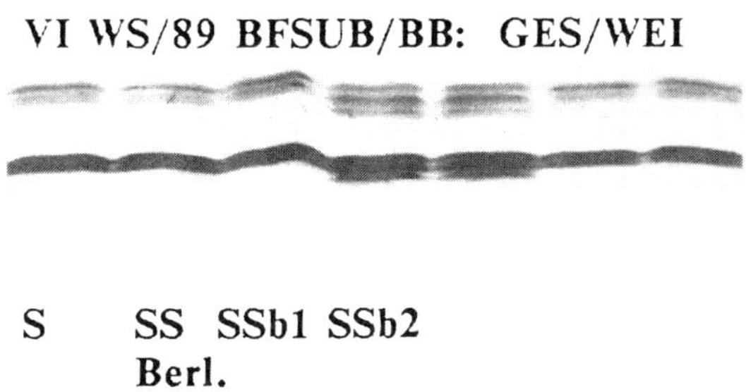

Table 2: **Nomenclature for the new variants ("subtypes") of factor B**

Designation[a]			
New	Old	Population	References
FB1	Fb1	Japanese	Nakamura et al. (*8*)
FB1	Fb1	Japanese	Suzuki et al. (*9*)
FB2	FB1	German	Geserick et al (*10*)
SB1	Sb1	German	Weidinger et al. (*11*)
SB2	Sb2	German	Weidinger et al. (*11*)
SB3	S_{Berlin}	German	Geserick et al. (*12*)

[a] The alphanumeric designation marks the position of the variant bands (B = *b*asic; different numbers for different positions).

Old and new nomenclatures for BF*F subtypes and their references are given below:

New:	FA	FB (*1*)
Old:	Fb	Fa (*5*)
	F'	F''

Rare variants ("subtypes") of BF F and S. Typing of many samples from different populations by IEF or by modified AGE has led to the discovery of new variants, all of them with cathodal (= basic) migration patterns. The variants will not be detected by means of standard AGE. Since their occurrence is rare (below or around 1%), the term "variant" is appropriate, facilitating their differentiation from the common "subtypes". The F variants ("Fb1" and "FB1") and the S variants ("Sb1", "Sb2" and "S Berlin") have proved to be different from each other (Fig. 2). The designations agreed upon during the Workshop are listed in Table 2.

Rare variants described as "BF Q0". In samples from three families with an assumed BF*Q0 allele, new and unexpected gene products were demonstrable. In all cases, the abnormal gene product has shown a faint protein band on separation of NANA'se-treated sera following IEF on agarose. Using a haemolytic overlap (*13*) this band has proved to be functionally active. The low protein concentration suggests a hyposynthetic variant. Therefore the designation "QL" was chosen to characterize its lower concentration. The additional capitals mark the electrophoretic position of the abnormal protein band: "S" for the position of the normal S band, and "M" for an intermediate, not yet definable position up to now (Table 3).

Methods for BF typing

Methods are available for typing the major BF variants by immunofixation AGE (*2*, *15*), for determining the relative migration distances (*3*); and for

Table 3: **New designations for abnormal BF gene products**

Designation		
New	Old	References
SQL	"BF*Q0"	Bertrams & Mauff (*14*)
M1QL	"BF*Q0"	Abbal et al. (unpublished)
M2QL	"BF*Q0"	Du Toit et al. (unpublished)

detecting the functional activity in haemolytic overlays (*13*).

BF subtypes and subtype "variants" may be detected in native, unconverted factor B, in the Ba fragment and/or the Bb fragment (*16* and Fig. 1a and 1b).

References

1. **Geserick, G. & Patzelt, D.** Factor B (BF) subtyping by isoelectric focusing: methods, nomenclatures, genetics and forensic application. *Electrophoresis*, **8**: 393–397 (1988).
2. **Alper, C.A. et al.** Genetic polymorphism in human glycine-rich beta-glycoprotein. *J. exp. med.*, **135**: 68–80 (1972).
3. **Mauff, G. et al.** The nomenclature of properdin factor B allotypes. *Z. Immunitätsforsch.*, **154**: 115–120 (1978).
4. **Mauff, G.** Application of the MHC-class III complement markers to population genetics. In: Ohayon, E. & Cambon-Thomsen, E., ed. *Human population genetics (INSERM)*, **142**: 143–166 (1986).
5. **Teng, Y.S. & Tan, S.G.** Subtyping of properdin factor B ("Bf") by isoelectrofocusing. *Hum. hered.*, **32**: 362–366 (1982).
6. **Geserick, G. et al.** Isoelectrofocusing in the study of the Bf system: existence of two common subtypes of the Bf allele. *Vox sang.*, **44**: 178–182 (1983).
7. **Abbal, M. et al.** Two subtypes of BF isolectrofocusing: differential linkage to other HLA markers. *Hum. genet.*, **69**: 181–183 (1987)
8. **Nakamura, S. et al.** A new BF F variant detected by polyacrylamide gel isoelectric focusing. *Hum. genet.*, **77**: 295–296 (1987).
9. **Suzuki, K. et al.** Subtyping of factor B by agarose gel electrophoresis. *Electrophoresis*, **6**: 481–485 (1987).
10. **Geserick, G. et al.** Detection of a new BF F subtype variant by isoelectric focusing. *Exp. clin. immunogenet.*, **6**: 156–161 (1989).
11. **Weidinger, S. et al.** Two new Bf S subtypes revealed by isolectric focusing and immunofixation. *Hum. genet.*, **68**: 90–92 (1984).
12. **Geserick, G. et al.** [Evidence for a "new" BF variant (BF Berlin) by isoelectric focusing.] *Biomed. biochim. acta*, **43**: 257–259 (1984) (in German).
13. **Mauff, G. et al.** A hemolytically inactive gene product of properdin factor B. *Immunobiol.*, **158**: 96–100 (1980).
14. **Bertrams, J. & Mauff, G.** Another family with a silent allele of properdin factor B polymorphism (BF*Q0). *Hum. genet.*, **70**: 321–323 (1985).
15. **Mauff, G. et al.** Properdin factor B (glycin-rich beta-glycoprotein or C3 proactivator)-polymorphism: genetic and biochemical aspects. First application to paternity cases. *Z. Immuno-Forsch. (Immunobiol.)*, **150**: 327–338 (1975).
16. **Siemens, I. et al.** The BF F subtypes are detectable in the Ba fragment of factor B. *Forensic science int.*, **42**: 279–286 (1989).

Nomenclature for secreted regulatory proteins of the immune system (interleukins)*

WHO–IUIS Nomenclature Subcommittee on Interleukin Designation[1]

The recommended procedures and criteria for interleukin designations are described. The offically adopted designations are, in sequence, from interleukin-1 to interleukin-10, including interleukin-1α and interleukin-1*β*.

Criteria for designations

The following procedures are recommended by a Subcommittee of the Nomenclature Committee of the International Union of Immunological Societies (IUIS) for the naming of new secreted regulatory proteins of the immune system (i.e., lymphokines, cytokines, interleukins). If the discoverers of such a molecule wish to utilize an interleukin designation (i.e., interleukin-n), they are urged not to do so unilaterally but to apply to the newly established Standing Committee on Interleukin Designation of IUIS for approval.[a] The granting of such an interleukin designation would depend on whether the following criteria have been met:

(1) The molecule shall have been purified, molecularly cloned and expressed. Its nucleotide and inferred amino acid sequence should be distinct from any currently known interleukin or indeed from any other already described molecule. The availability of monoclonal antibodies that may neutralize its function would be desirable but not absolutely required, as would information regarding the chromosomal location of the gene encoding the molecule.

(2) The molecule shall have been shown to be a natural product of cells of the immune system, to mediate a potentially important function in immune responses, and preferably also to have more than a single function so that a simple functional name might not be adequate. It is preferred if it could be shown that the predominant actions of the molecule were to mediate functions in the immune system, but it is recognized that this may be difficult to establish. The terms "immune system" and "immune responses" shall be defined very broadly to include leukocytes other than lymphocytes and monocytes as important participants.

(3) If the molecule is a member of an already characterized family of molecules that have their major functions outside the immune system, it would be preferable in most circumstances to use a designation consistent with the naming of other members of the family rather than adopting an interleukin designation.

(4) The Subcommittee in no way wishes to discourage the use of descriptive names for new lymphokines and cytokines. Indeed, it generally recommends that interleukin designations only be sought when the discoverers or other major participants in the field have a compelling reason for seeking such a name. Well-chosen descriptive or

---

* This article was drafted by a group of experts working under the auspices of the International Union of Immunological Societies (IUIS) and has been approved by the Nomenclature Committee of IUIS. A French translation appears on pages 485–486. Requests for reprints and all correspondence should be addressed to the Chairman of the IUIS Nomenclature Committee, Dr Michel Kazatchkine, Unité d'Immunopathologie, Hôpital Broussais, 96 rue Didot, 75014 Paris, France.

[1] Members of the Nomenclature Subcommittee: W.E. Paul (USA) (*Chairman*), Tadamitsu Kishimoto (Japan), F. Melchers (Switzerland), D. Metcalf (Australia), T. Mosmann (Canada), J. Oppenheim (USA), Nancy Ruddle (USA), and J. Van Snick (Belgium).

[a] Standing Committee on Interleukin Designation: Chairman: T. Mosmann, Department of Immunology, University of Alberta, Canada.

Reprint No. **5199**

functional names may have mnemonic value that an interleukin designation is likely to lack.

Based on the proposed requirements for the award of an interleukin designation, it is very unlikely that such a designation could be granted prior to the initial publication describing a new factor. Thus, even if the authors wish that an interleukin designation be awarded, they are urged to choose some provisional name. If they wish, they may indicate in their publications that they intend to apply for an interleukin designation, without specifying what that designation may be.

In a situation in which more than a single research group was involved in the discovery of the molecule or in some very important aspects of the characterization of the molecule, it is desirable that agreement be obtained from all the major contributors prior to the application for an interleukin designation. If an interleukin designation is sought for a molecule that has been studied by several groups for an extended period of time, it is likely that the Standing Committee will recommend that some type of consensus on the part of all concerned be obtained prior to application for an interleukin designation.

The Standing Committee may wish to obtain expert advice regarding the suitability of awarding an interleukin designation to a particular molecule. Accordingly, supporting material regarding the characterization of the potential interleukin must be in the public domain and, preferably, should have been published in refereed journals.

Designations

A list of official interleukin designations will be sent to journals that regularly publish papers in this field. The editors will be asked to request their authors not to use non-official interleukin designations. Indeed, once this mechanism is in place, the immunological community is strongly urged not to unilaterally adopt interleukin designations in order to avoid the confusion that may occur when several molecules are given the same designation or when molecules whose principal functions lie outside the immune system receive an interleukin designation.

Currently accepted interleukin designations officially adopted by the IUIS Nomenclature Committee are listed below:

Interleukin-1 α ; Interleukin-1 β
Interleukin-2
Interleukin-3
Interleukin-4
Interleukin-5
Interleukin-6
Interleukin-7
Interleukin-8
Interleukin-9
Interleukin-10.

Nomenclature for secreted regulatory proteins of the immune system (interleukins): update*

IUIS/WHO Nomenclature Committee[1]

The officially adopted designations for interleukins now include IL-11, IL-12 and IL-13, in addition to the previously recommended IL-1 to IL-10, including IL-1α and IL-1β.

The criteria that should be met by a newly described secreted regulatory protein of the immune system in order for it to be granted an interleukin designation were defined by a IUIS/WHO Nomenclature Subcommittee in 1991 (*Bulletin of the World Health Organization*, 1991, **69**: 483–484). The officially adopted designations at that time were from interleukin-1 to interleukin-10, including interleukin-1α and interleukin-1β.

It is now recommended that the designations IL-11, IL-12 and IL-13 be adopted. The molecules have been fully characterized on a molecular level and shown to exhibit distinct regulatory functions in the immune system.

Authors describing a new factor who wish to utilize an interleukin designation are urged not to do so unilaterally but to apply to the IUIS/WHO Standing Committee on Interleukin Designation for approval (see footnote 1).

* A French translation appears on page 812. Requests for reprints should be addressed to the Chairman of the IUIS Nomenclature Committee, Professor Michel D. Kazatchkine, Service d'Immunologie, Hôpital Broussais, 96 rue Didot, 75014 Paris, France.

[1] Standing Committee on Interleukin Designation (*Chairman*: Professor T. Kishimoto, Osaka Medical School, Osaka, Japan. Fax, 81-06-879-3839).

Reprint No. **5534**

Interleukin 16 (IL-16)*

IUIS/WHO Standing Committee on Interleukin Designation[1]

Interleukin 16 was originally known as lymphocyte chemoattractant factor (LCF) (*1*, *2*) because of its first identified function. In its biologically active form, it is a cationic homotetramer consisting of 14 kDa chains (*2*, *3*). It has a unique cDNA that codes for a 130 amino acid protein, which is unrelated to previously described chemokines or other chemotactic/growth factor cytokines (*3*). The gene is located on chromosome 15. All of IL-16's biological activities depend upon the cell surface expression of CD4 (*3–6*) through which it transmits its functional signals (*5*, *7*) independently of the expression of CD3 (*4–7*). In this regard, it is a CD4 ligand. As a result, $CD4^+$ T cells, eosinophils (*6*), and monocytes (*4*) are responsive, while $CD4^-$ cells are not.

In addition to its chemotactic activity, IL-16 activates resting $CD4^+$ T cells, as indicated by upregulation of HLA-DR antigen and IL-2R (CD25) expression. A result of IL-16-dependent CD25 expression (*4*) is a G_0 to G_1 cell cycle phase shift that defines an IL-2 responsive competence point (*3*) associated with reversible unresponsiveness to antigen (*8*).

IL-16 is a chemotactic and activating factor for $CD4^+$ monocytes, in which it induces HLA-DR expression via a CD4-dependent, interferon-independent pathway (*4*). It is one of the most potent chemotactic factors for eosinophils (*6*). IL-16 was first identified as a product of $CD8^+$ T cells (*9*), in which it is constitutively synthesized and stored in a biologically active preformed state (*10*). $CD4^+$ T cells, bronchial epithelial cells (*11*), and eosinophils are additional sources. Secretion of IL-16 can be induced from peripheral blood mononuclear cells by antigen (*1*), concanavalin A (1) and histamine (*9*, *10*) and from epithelial cells by histamine (*11*).

Murine and rat homologue proteins have been identified (*12*); however their cDNAs have not been cloned. IL-16 has been identified as an early chemoattractant/growth factor in the bronchoalveolar lavage of antigen-challenged atopic asthmatics (*13*); in the bronchoalveolar lavage of patients with sarcoidosis; and in the blister fluid of patients with bullous pemphigoid (*14*) — all diseases associated with a $CD4^+$ T cell organ infiltration.

References

1. **Center DM, Cruikshank W.** Modulation of lymphocyte migration by human lymphokines. I. Identification and characterization of chemoattractant activity for lymphocytes from mitogen-stimulated mononuclear cells. *Journal of immunology*, 1982, **128**: 2563–2568.
2. **Cruikshank W, Center DM.** Modulation of lymphocyte migration by human lymphokines. II. Purification of a lymphotactic factor (LCF). *Journal of immunology*, 1982, **128**: 2569–2571.
3. **Cruikshank WW et al.** Molecular and functional analysis of A lymphocyte chemoattractant factor: association of biologic function with CD4 expression. *Proceedings of the National Academy Sciences of the USA*, 1994, **91**: 5109–5113.
4. **Cruikshank WW et al.** Lymphokine activation of T4+ lymphocytes and monocytes. *Journal of immunology*, 1987, **138**: 3817.
5. **Cruikshank WW et al.** Lymphocyte chemoattractant factor (LCF) induces CD4-dependent intracytoplasmic signalling in lymphocytes. *Journal of immunology*, 1991, **146**: 2928–2934.
6. **Rand T et al.** CD4-Mediated stimulation of human eosinophils: lymphocyte chemoattractant factor and other CD4-binding ligands elicit eosinophil migration. *Journal of experimental medicine*, 1991, **173**: 1521–1528.
7. **Ryan T, Cruikshank WW, Center DM.** Activation of CD4 associated p56 lck by the lymphocyte chemoattractant factor. Dissociation of kinase enzymatic activity with chemotactic response. *Journal of biological chemistry*, in press.

* Requests for reprints should be addressed to the Chairman of the IUIS/WHO Nomenclature Committee: Professor Michel D. Kazatchkine, Service d'Immunologie, Hôpital Broussais, 96 rue Didot, 75014 Paris, France.

[1] Chairman: Professor T. Kishimoto, Japan.

Reprint No. **5725**

8. **Theodore AC et al.** Suppression of the immune response by a natural CD4-dependent interleukin. *American journal of respiratory and critical care medicine*, 1995, **151**: 452A.
9. **Center DM et al.** Functional characteristics of histamine receptor-bearing mononuclear cells. I. Selective production of lymphocyte chemoattractant lymphokine-utilizing histamine as a ligand. *Journal of immunology*, 1983, **131**: 1856–1859.
10. **Laberge S et al.** Mechanism of histamine induced lymphocyte chemoattractant factor release from CD8+ T cells. *Journal of immunology* (in press).
11. **Bellini A et al.** Bronchial epithelial cells of patients with asthma release chemoattractant factors for T lymphocytes. *Journal of allergy and clinical immunology*, 1993, **92**: 412–424.
12. **McFadden RG, Vickers KE.** Rat lymphokines control migration of non-sensitized lymphocytes. *Cellular immunology*, 1989, **118**: 345–357.
13. **Cruikshank WW et al.** Identification of lymphocyte chemoattractant activities following antigen challenge of atopic asthmatics. *American journal of respiratory cell and molecular biology*, in press.
14. **Center DM, Wintroub BU, Austen KF.** Identification of chemoattractant activity for lymphocytes in blister fluid of patients with bullous pemphigoid: evidence for the presence of a lymphokine. *Journal of investigative dermatology*, 1983, **81**: 204–208.

Nomenclature for secreted regulatory proteins of the immune system (Interleukins): update*

IUIS/WHO Standing Committee on Interleukin Designation[1]

The officially adopted designations for interleukins now include IL-14 and IL-15, in addition to the previously recommended IL-1 to IL-13 and IL-16.

The criteria that should be met by a newly described secreted regulatory protein of the immune system in order for it to be granted an interleukin designation were defined by the IUIS/WHO Nomenclature Subcommittee in 1991 (*1*). At that time the officially adopted designations were for interleukin-1 to interleukin-10, including interleukin-1α and interleukin-1β.

Subsequently it was recommended that the designations IL-11, IL-12 and IL-13 be adopted (*2*) and it is now proposed that the designations IL-14 and IL-15 also be adopted. Both IL-14 and IL-15 have been fully characterized at the molecular level and shown to exhibit distinct regulatory functions in the immune system. Also a separate recommendation concerning IL-16 has recently been published (*3*).

Workers describing a new factor using an interleukin designation are urged not to do so unilaterally but to apply to the Chairman of the IUIS/WHO Standing Committee on Interleukin Designation for approval.

References

1. **IUIS/WHO Nomenclature Committee on Interleukin Designation.** Nomenclature for secreted regulatory proteins of the immune system (interleukins). *Bulletin of the World Health Organization*, 1991, **69**: 483–484.
2. **IUIS/WHO Nomenclature Committee on Interleukin Designation.** Nomenclature for secreted regulatory proteins of the immune system (interleukins): update. *Bulletin of the World Health Organization*, 1994, **72**: 811
3. **IUIS/WHO Nomenclature Committee on Interleukin Designation.** Interleukin 16 (IL-16). *Bulletin of the World Health Organization*, 1996, **74**: 451–452.

* Requests for reprints should be addressed to the Chairman of the IUIS Nomenclature Committee: Professor M.W. Turner, Immunobiology Unit, Institute of Child Health, 30 Guilford Street, London WC1N 1EH, England.

[1] Chairman, IUIS/WHO Standing Committee on Interleukin Designation: Professor T. Kishimoto, Osaka University Medical School, Osaka, Japan.

Reprint No. **5767**

Nomenclature for clusters of differentiation (CD) of antigens defined on human leukocyte populations*

IUIS-WHO NOMENCLATURE SUBCOMMITTEE[1]

Evaluation of 139 monoclonal antibodies detecting human leukocyte differentiation antigens during the First International Workshop on Human Leucocyte Differentiation Antigens in 1982 permitted the designation of a nomenclature for the Clusters of Differentiation of antigens defined on human leukocyte populations.

The general principles of this nomenclature, as well as the characteristics of the fifteen Clusters of Differentiation which have so far been defined, are presented.

In November 1982, the results of the First International Workshop on Human Leucocyte Differentiation Antigens, sponsored by the International Union of Immunological Societies (IUIS), Institut national de la Santé et de la Recherche médicale (INSERM), the Medical Research Council, and WHO, were presented at a meeting held in Paris. The data from these common blind studies were collected by 55 research groups from 14 different countries for publication.[a] A total of 139 monoclonal antibodies were examined in immunofluorescence tests and the results expressed as a percentage of positive cells. The statistical analysis relied on the distances between antibodies. The distance between 2 antibodies for a given target cell type is the average of the absolute difference between the reactivities of the 2 antibodies for all target cells of the type considered. Then cluster analysis of the matrix of distances between all pairs of antibodies and algorithmic computation permitted the definition of groups of antibodies that were similar, and those that were clearly different, on each type of target cell.

The clusters of differentiation were then readily delineated from summing-up tables of groups of antibodies obtained for each target cell type; these clusters included the antibodies that always had very similar reactivities. Moreover, the confrontation between blind studies on the relative molecular mass ("molecular weight"), performed with the antibodies, and cluster analysis showed an almost perfect correspondence. These final clusters were termed *clusters of differentiation* (CD) following the general recommendations (Table 1) adopted by the Nomenclature Subcommittee, which were approved with no objections or comments from the 250 scientists (including most of the workshop participants) at the Paris meeting mentioned above.

Both oral and written designations of the first eleven clusters (as shown in Table 2) were officially adopted by the Nomenclature Subcommittee which met in Kyoto in August 1983 during the Vth International Congress of Immunology.

The new nomenclature relies on a simple, unambiguous, and adaptable system, thus avoiding the major difficulties in communication which had previously arisen from the multiplicity of nomenclatures used. It is the one that should now be followed.

*

* *

A. Bernard, Institut Gustave Roussy, Villejuif, France

I. Bernstein, Fred Hutchison Cancer Research Center, Seattle, WA, USA

* A French translation of this terminology note appears on pages 813-815.

[1] See pages 809-810 for the names of the members of this Committee. Requests for reprints should be sent to Dr S.F. Schlossman, 44 Binney Street, Boston, MA 02115, USA.

[a] BERNARD, A. ET AL., ed., *Leucocyte typing. Report of the First International Workshop on Human Leucocyte Differentiation Antigens*. Heidelberg, Springer Verlag, 1984, pp. 9–143.

L. Boumsell, Hôpital Saint-Louis, Paris, France
J. Dausset, Hôpital Saint-Louis, Paris, France
R. Evans, Sloan Kettering Research Institute, New York, NY, USA
J. Hansen, Fred Hutchison Cancer Research Center, Seattle, WA, USA
B. Haynes, Duke University Medical Center, Durham, NC, USA
J. Kersey, University Hospitals and Clinics, Minneapolis, MN, USA
W. Knapp, Institut für Immunologie, Vienna, Austria
A. McMichael, John Radcliffe Hospital, Oxford, England
C. Milstein, MRC Laboratory of Molecular Biology, Cambridge, England
E. Reinherz, Dana Farber Cancer Center, Boston, MA, USA
R.E. Ritts, Mayo Research Foundation, Rochester, NY, USA
S.F. Schlossman, Dana Farber Cancer Center, Boston, MA, USA

Table 1. Explanation of the nomenclature system for leukocyte differentiation antigens

CD No. [cell, M.W.] name of monoclonal antibody

CD: Cluster of differentiation.
No. Here is given the number officially ascribed to the cluster.[a]

In square brackets:

Cell: Typical cell of the particular CD, or cell type on which the relative molecular mass or "molecular weight" (M.W.) was determined.

M.W.: "Molecular weight" or relative molecular mass of the antigen on the particular cell type, as determined on the specimen reduced in a strong denaturant. The M.W. is preceded by:
gp: glycoprotein
gl: glycolipid
cho: carbohydrate
When the M.W. is not known, the letter "u" (= unknown) is used in its place.

After the brackets:

The name of the particular monoclonal antibody is mentioned here.
Example: CALLA,[b] investigated by the monoclonal antibody J5 on non-T, non-B leukaemic cells, should be designated:
CD10 [nT–nB, gp100] J5
Oral designation should be limited to CD10.

[a] Whenever definitive official recognition of a given CD cannot be achieved, but it is nevertheless felt that an official designation should be provisionally adopted, the CD could be termed CDw No. In Kyoto (August 1983), the Subcommittee officially recognized 11 CDs and provisionally termed 4 additional CDws. Their identity and designation are indicated in Table 2.

[b] CALLA: the former common acute lymphoblastic leukaemia antigen.

Table 2. Clusters of differentiation of human leukocyte differentiation antigens

Cluster designation[a]	Antibodies[b]	Typical leukocyte subpopulations	Leukocyte malignancies[c]
CD1 [Thy, gp45,12]	NA1/34, T6, M241, D47	Corticothymocytes	Few[d] T-ALL and T-LL
CD2 [T, gp50]	9.6, T11, 35.1	All T-cells forming E rosette	Most [d] T-cell malignancies
CD3 [T, gp19-29]	T3, UCHT 1, 89bl, 38.1	Mature T-cells	Most T-CLL and CTCL Few T-ALL and T-LL
CD4 [T, gp56–62]	T4, Leu3a, 91D6	Subset of T-cells Mostly inducers	Few T-ALL, some[d] T-CLL Most CTCL
CD5 [T, gp67]	A50, 10.2, T1, UCHT2, SC1, AMG4, T101, Cris 1, H65, HH9	Pan T + subpopulation B-cells	Most T-cell malignancies Some B-CLL
CD6 [T, gp120]	12.1, T411, B614, WT31, MBG6	Mature T + subpopulation B-cells	Few T-ALL, most T-CLL and CTCL. Some B-CLL
CD7 [T, gp41]	3A1, 4A, CL1.3	Pan T	Most T-ALL, some T-CLL Few CTCL
CD8 [T, gp32-33]	Leu2a, T8, M236, 51.1, UCHT4, 2D2, B9.4.1, B9.3.1, B9.7.6, B9.2.4, B9.8.6, B9.11.10, B9.1.1, C10, T811	Subset of T-cells Mostly cytotoxic/suppressor	Few T-ALL and T-CLL

Table 2. — *continued*

Cluster designation[a]	Antibodies[b]	Typical leukocyte subpopulations	Leukocyte malignancies[c]
CD9 [nT-nB, gp24]	BA2, DU-ALL-1, FMC8, SJ9A-4, WB3	Monocytes	Most nonT-nonB ALL Few B-CLL
CD10 [nT-nB, gp100]	J5, BA3, NL-1, 24.1, VIL-A1	Pre-B cell Polymorphs	Most nonT-nonB ALL
CD11 [M, G, u]	MO1, B2.12, M522	Monocytes and granulocytes Some bone marrow cells	Some M4 and most M5 stages of AML. Some CML
CDw12 [M, G, u]	20.2, M67	Monocytes and granulocytes	Few M4 and M5 stages of AML
CDw13 [M, G, u]	MY7, DU-HL60-4, MCS.2	Monocytes and granulocytes	Most M1 and few M4 or M5 stages of AML. Some CML
CDw14 [M, u]	20.3, 5F1, MOP15, MO2, MOS1, MY4, MOS39, TM18, MOP9, FMC17	Monocytes	Few M4 and some M5 stages of AML
CDw15 [G, u]	80H3, B13.9, MCS.1, 82H7 FMC12, FMC13, WM37, DU-HL60-1, FMC10, WM27, WM30, G1120, TG8, WM38, TG1, DU-HL60-3, G2, B4.3, VIMD5, WM41, 1G10	Granulocytes Some bone marrow cells	Most M4 and some M5 stages of AML. Some CML

[a] See Table 1.

[b] List of antibodies in the cluster.

[c] Abbreviations used:
- ALL, acute lymphoblastic leukaemia
- LL, lymphoblastic lymphoma
- CLL, chronic lymphocytic leukaemia
- CTCL, cutaneous T-cell lymphoma
- AML, acute myeloblastic leukaemia
- CML, chronic myelogenous leukaemia.

[d] Frequency of positive cases is indicated as:
"few" for frequency of 10–39%
"some" for frequency of 40–70%
"most" for frequency of > 70%

CD antigens 1993: an updated nomenclature for clusters of differentiation on human cells*

IUIS/WHO Subcommittee on CD Nomenclature[1]

The 5th International Workshop on Human Leukocyte Differentiation Antigens (Boston, USA, 3–7 November 1993) recommended the adoption of 48 new CD clusters and subclusters and the redefinition of 14 previously established clusters. The additions and changes made to the existing CD nomenclature are summarized in a Table.

Introduction

The nomenclature for clusters of differentiation (CD), which is dedicated to the designation of cell surface structures of human cells, was established by the International Workshop on Human Leukocyte Differentiation Antigens and continues to be updated by these Workshops. The CD nomenclature was initially proposed to cluster monoclonal antibodies (mAbs) of different sources that recognize the same human leukocyte differentiation antigen. The nomenclature is based on analysis of the results of blinded studies of the molecular mass of antigens recognized by mAbs submitted for evaluation to the Workshop and of the reactivity of the mAbs with target cells. The nomenclature was aimed to be simple, unambiguous and adaptable.

The CD nomenclature is now widely used to designate the molecular species recognized by a mAb. New mAbs are characterized and therefore new CD antigens are defined after each International Workshop. In addition, the CDw ("Workshop") designation is attributed to either (1) a single mAb recognizing the cell surface product of a transfected gene, or (2) a new molecule identified by one or two mAbs generated in the same laboratory. The CD # R symbols are given to indicate that the tissue distribution of CD # may be restricted. In some cases the restriction has been attributed to alternative splicing; in the latter instance, the letter R is followed by a letter corresponding to relevant exons.

Results

The results of the 5th International Workshop on Human Leukocyte Differentiation Antigens were presented on 3–7 November 1993 at a meeting in Boston, MA, USA. The participants represented the efforts of more than 500 laboratories worldwide, which joined together over a two-year period to analyse 1450 antibodies and characterize over 150 molecules. Blind panels for all monoclonal antibodies (mAbs), every CD antigen, every known candidate for CD status, and all mAbs of undefined specificity were analysed by flow cytometry. Other dedicated laboratories undertook serological, molecular, biochemical and histochemical characterization of the mAbs and the structures they defined. The results obtained by all groups showed almost perfect concordance.

Detailed results of these studies will be published separately.[a] In addition, a Leukocyte Differentiation Antigen Database (LDAD) has been developed to (1) provide identifying information on all molecules and mAbs studied in the Workshop, and (2) display/analyse the quantitative expression of each molecule on more than 80 cell types.[b] Based on these findings, the Workshop recommends the adoption of 48 new CD clusters and subclusters and the redefinition of 14 previously established clusters. The additions and changes made to the existing CD nomenclature are summarized in Table 1.

---

* This report has been approved by the IUIS/WHO Nomenclature Committee. A résumé in French appears on page 808. Requests for reprints should be addressed to the Chairman of the IUIS Nomenclature Committee, Professor Michel Kazatchkine, Unité d'Immunologie, Hôpital Broussais, 96 rue Didot, 75014 Paris, France.

[1] The Subcommittee's members are S.F. Schlossmann (*Chairman*), L. Boumsell, W. Gilks, J.M. Harlan, T. Kishimoto, C. Morimoto, J. Ritz, S. Shaw, R.L. Silverstein, T.A. Springer, T.F. Tedder and R.F. Todd.

Reprint No. **5532**

[a] **Schlossmann SF et al.**, eds. *White cell differentiation antigens.* Oxford, Oxford University Press, 1994 (in press).

[b] The LDAD program runs on IBM PCs and via emulation on Macintosh. It may be downloaded freely via anonymous ftp from balrog.nci.nih.gov (156.40.182.2) or purchased on disk (inquiries by fax 301–480–2052).

Table 1: **CD antigens 1993**

CD Designation	Common name	Workshop section	Mol. mass reduced
CD15s	sLe^x, Sialyl Lewis ^{x}	Adhesion	
CD16	FcR IIIA/FcR IIIB	Myeloid	50–65
CD16b	FcR IIIB	Myeloid	48
CD32	Previously CDw32, FcRII	Myeloid	40
CD42a	GPIX	Platelets	23
CD42b	GPIB, α	Platelets	135,23
CD42c	GP1B-β	Platelets	22
CD42d	GPV	Platelets	85
CD44	Pgp-1	Adhesion	80–90
CD44R	Restricted epitope on CD44	Adhesion	
CD49a	VLA-1, α1 integrin chain	Adhesion	210
CD49b	VLA-2, α2 integrin chain	Adhesion	160
CD49c	VLA-3, α3 integrin chain	Adhesion	125
CD49d	VLA-4, α4 integrin chain	Adhesion	150,80,70
CD49e	VLA-5, α5 integrin chain	Adhesion	135,25
CD49f	VLA-6, α6 integrin chain	Adhesion	120,25
CD50	ICAM-3	Adhesion	124
CD51/ CD61	Complex dependent epitope	Adhesion	
CD52	Campath-1	Blind	21–28
CD62E	E-selectin, ELAM-1	Adhesion	115
CD62L	L-selectin, LAM-1, TQ-1	Adhesion	75–80
CD62P	P-selectin, GMP-140, PADGEM	Adhesion	150
CD66a	BGP	Myeloid	180–200
CD66b	CD67, p100, CGM6	Myeloid	95–100
CD66c	NCA	Myeloid	90–95
CD66d	CGM1	Myeloid	30
CD66e	CEA, carcinoembryonic antigen	Myeloid	180–200
CD67	Now CD66b		
CD70	CD27-ligand	Activation	55,75,95, 110,170
CDw76	Previously CD76	B Cell	NA
CD79a	mb-1, Igα	B Cell	33,40
CD79b	B29, Igβ	B Cell	33,40
CD80	B7, BB1	B Cell	60
CD81	TAPA-1	B Cell	22
CD82	R2, IA4, 4F9	B Cell	50–53
CD83	HB15	B Cell	43
CDw84		B Cell	73
CD85	VMP-55, GH1/75	B Cell	120,83
CD86	FUN-1, BU63	B Cell	80
CD87	UPA-R	Myeloid	50–65
CD88	C5aR	Myeloid	42
CD89	FcαR	Myeloid	55–75
CDw90	Thy-1	Myeloid	25–35
CD91	α_2M-R	Myeloid	600
CDw92		Myeloid	70
CD93		Myeloid	120
CD94	KP43	NK Cell	43
CD95	APO-1, FAS	Activation	42
CD96	TACTILE	Activation	160
CD97		Activation	74,80,89
CD98	4F2, 2F3	T Cell	80,40
CD99	E2, MIC2	T Cell	32
CD99R	CD99 mAb restricted	T Cell	32
CD100	BB18, A8	T Cell	150
CDw101	BB27, BA27	T Cell	140
CD102	ICAM-2	Adhesion	60
CD103	HML-1	Adhesion	150,25
CD104	β4 integrin chain	Adhesion	220
CD105	Endoglin	Endothelial	95
CD106	VCAM-1, INCAM-110	Endothelial	100,110
CD107a	LAMP-1	Platelet	110
CD107b	LAMP-2	Platelet	120
CDw108		Adhesion	80
CDw109	8A3, 7D1	Endothelial	170,150
CD115	CSF-1R; M-CSFR	Myeloid	150
CDw116	HGM-CSFR, GM-CSFR	Cytokine	75–85
CD117	SCFR, cKIT	Cytokine	145
CDw119	IFNγR	Cytokine	90
CD120a	TNFR;55kD	Cytokine	55
CD120b	TNFR;75kD	Cytokine	75
CDw121a	IL-1R;Type1	Cytokine	80
CDw121b	IL-1R;Type2	Cytokine	68
CD122	IL-2R;75kD, IL-2Rβ	Cytokine	75
CDw124	IL-4R	Cytokine	140
CD126	IL-6R	Cytokine	80
CDw127	IL-7R	Cytokine	75
CDw128	IL-8R	Cytokine	57–67
CDw130	IL-6R-GP130SIG	Cytokine	130

CD antigens 1996: updated nomenclature for clusters of differentiation on human cells*

IUIS/WHO Subcommittee on CD Nomenclature[1]

The 6th International Workshop on Human Leukocyte Differentiation Antigens, held in Kobe, Japan, on 10–14 November 1996, recommended the adoption of 41 new CD clusters and subclusters and the redefinition of 20 previously established clusters. The additions and changes are summarized in tabular form in this article.

The nomenclature for clusters of differentiation (CD), which is dedicated to the designation of cell surface structures of human cells, was established by the International Workshop on Human Leukocyte Differentiation Antigens, and was last updated in 1993 (*1*). The nomenclature is based on analysis of the results of blinded studies of the molecular mass of antigens recognized by cluster monoclonal antibodies (mAbs) submitted for evaluation to the Workshop and of the reactivity of the mAbs with target cells.

The results of the 6th International Workshop on Human Leukocyte Differentiation Antigens were presented on 10–14 November 1996 at a conference held in Kobe, Japan. More than 500 laboratories worldwide participated in the evaluation of 1152 antibodies and in the characterization of over 190 molecules over a 2-year period. The serological, molecular, biochemical, histochemical, and functional characterization of the mAbs and the structures defined by them were carried out by dedicated participating laboratories. The cross-lineage blind panels for all mAbs, including every CD, every known candidate for CD status, and all mAbs of undefined specificity, were analysed using flow cytometry and the results of the blind panel study analysed statistically to identify possible antibody clusters. The results obtained by all the groups showed almost perfect concordance. Detailed results of these Workshop studies will be published separately (*2*). Concise summaries ("CD guides") for each of the 190 molecules considered at the Workshop have also been prepared and are undergoing peer review.[a] In addition, the Workshop database has been made available on the World Wide Web server to provide identifying information on all molecules and mAbs studied at the Workshop and to display and analyse the quantitative expression of each molecule on more than 70 cell types used for the cross-lineage blind panel study.[b] Based on these findings, the Workshop organizers recommended the adoption of 41 new CD clusters and subclusters and the redefinition of 20 previously established clusters. Table 1 summarizes the additions and changes made to the existing CD nomenclature.

---

* This report has been approved by the IUIS/WHO Nomenclature Committee. A résumé in French appears on page 387. Requests for reprints should be addressed to the Chairman of the IUIS Nomenclature Committee, Professor M.W. Turner, Immunobiology Unit, Institute of Child Health, 30 Guilford Street, London WC1N 1EH, England.

[1] The Subcommittee's members are S.F. Schlossman (*Chairman*), L. Boumsell, T. Kishimoto, W. Knapp, D. Mason, A. McMichael, S. Shaw, T.A. Springer, T. Tedder, R. Todd, H. Waldman, and H. Zola.

Reprint No. **5793**

[a] These summaries are available on the World Wide Web at http://www.ncbi.nlm.nih.gov/prow. For information, send an e-mail request to prow@nih.gov.

[b] The Workshop's database is accessible on the World Wide Web at http://mol.genes.nig.ac.jp/hlda/. For information, send an e-mail request to hlda-master@ddbj.nig.ac.jp.

Table 1: **CD antigens 1996**

CD designation	Common name/remarks	Workshop Section
CD45RC	Restricted epitope of CD45	Non-lineage
CD52	CDw52	Non-lineage
CD65	CDw65	Myeloid
CD65s	Sialylated form of CD65	Myeloid
CD66f	PMG-1	Myeloid
CD84	CDw84	B cell
CD90	CDw90, Thy-1	Adhesion
CD101	CDw101	Myeloid
CD114	G-CSFR	Myeloid
CD109	CDw109	Endothelial
CD116	CDw116, GM-CSFR	Cytokine
CD121a	CDw121a, IL-1R; type 1	Cytokine
CDw123	IL-3Rα	Cytokine
CD124	CDw124, IL-4R	Cytokine
CDw125	IL-5Rα	Cytokine
CD127	CDw127, IL-7R	Cytokine
CD130	CDw130, IL-6R-gp130 signal transducer	Cytokine
CDw131	Common β	Cytokine
CD132	Common γ	Cytokine
CD134	OX40	Cytokine
CD135	Flt3, Flk2	Cytokine
CDw136	MSP-R, macrophage stimulating protein receptor	Cytokine
CDw137	4-1BB	Cytokine
CD138	Syndecan-1	B cell
CD139		B cell
CD140a	PDGFRα, platelet derived growth factor receptor	Endothelial
CD140b	PDGFRβ, platelet derived growth factor receptor	Endothelial
CD141	Thrombomodulin	Endothelial
CD142	Tissue factor	Endothelial
CD143	ACE, angiotensin converting enzyme	Endothelial
CD144	VE-cadherin	Endothelial
CDw145		Endothelial
CD146	MUC18, S-endo	Endothelial
CD147	Neurothelin, basigin	Endothelial
CD148	HPTP-eta, p260 phosphatase	Non-lineage
CDw149	MEM-133	Non-lineage
CDw150	SLAM, IPO-3	Non-lineage
CD151	PETA-3	Platelet
CD152	CTLA-4	T cell
CD153	CD30L, CD30 ligand	T cell
CD154	CD40L, CD40 ligand, T-BAM	T cell
CD155	PVR, poliovirus receptor	Myeloid
CD156	ADAM8, MS2(mouse homologue)	Myeloid
CD157	BST-1, MO-5	Myeloid
CD158a	p58.1, MHC class-I specific NK receptors	NK cell
CD158b	p58.2, MHC class-I specific NK receptors	NK cell
CD161	NKRP-1	NK cell
CD162	PSGL-1	Adhesion
CD163	M130	Myeloid
CD164	MGC-24	Adhesion
CD165	GP37/AD2	Adhesion
CD166	ALCAM	Adhesion

A proposal for the definition of terms related to locomotion of leukocytes and other cells*

There is currently much confusion of terms relating to locomotion of leukocytes and other cells. Standardized and precise use of terms is, however, indispensable for analysis of the basic mechanisms controlling such locomotion. The present proposal is intended to serve as a basis for a standardized system of reporting locomotor behaviour of leukocytes and other cells and their responses to environmental stimuli. Definitions of the terms random locomotion, directional locomotion, chemotaxis, chemokinesis, and intrinsic locomotor capacity are proposed. Examples are given to demonstrate the application of the terms in the experimental and clinical analysis of cell locomotion.

Active locomotion of cells or organisms depends on intrinsic cellular mechanisms, which are influenced by factors from the environment. A response to an environmental stimulus that takes the form of a directed orientation reaction is called *taxis*; one that takes the form of undirected locomotion is called *kinesis* (for review see *1*). The words *chemotaxis* (*2*) and *chemokinesis* (*3*) may be used to describe such reactions when the stimulus from the environment is chemical. Chemotaxis and chemokinesis play a considerable role in cell locomotion, particularly in leukocytes (*4–6*). Analysis of leukocyte locomotion in the presence of a source of a chemical attractant shows that these cells (*a*) become morphologically oriented in the concentration gradient and (*b*) migrate directionally towards the source of the gradient (*7*). Cells exposed to certain chemical stimuli in the absence of a gradient show enhanced locomotion, whose speed is determined by the stimulus although it is not directional (*8–11*). It remains to be evaluated whether and to what extent chemotaxis and chemokinesis can be mediated by identical factors. The capacity for active locomotion is a prerequisite for leukocyte emigration into inflammatory sites and influx of these cells into such sites may be regulated by changes in speed and/or directionality of the cells. Therefore, experimental tests of cell function must be capable of distinguishing these different modes of leukocyte locomotion. Present methods measure fairly complex phenomena, such as "random locomotion" and "directional locomotion". Further analysis of these complex phenomena will yield information on leukocyte functions and responses, such as intrinsic locomotor capacity, chemokinesis, or chemotaxis.

There is currently serious confusion of terms relating to locomotion of leukocytes. In particular, the term chemotaxis has been used in a variety of ways, so that it often becomes impossible to discern what the author had in mind. Frequently the term "chemotaxis" has been used interchangeably with "directional locomotion" or even to describe any form of movement of leukocytes (for instance into filters) in the presence of chemical substances (see *6*). The terms "random migration" or "random locomotion" have been used interchangeably to denote different qualities such as intrinsic locomotor capacity, changes in the speed of locomotion, or just undirected movement. The way the terms are used also varies in different fields of biology. For instance,

* The names of the scientists responsible for formulating this proposal will be found in the Annex. Reprints requests should be addressed to: Dr H. U. Keller, Institute of Pathology, Freiburgstrasse 30, CH-3010 Bern, Switzerland. A French version of this article will be published in a later issue of the *Bulletin*.

the word chemotaxis means one thing for those who study locomotion of bacteria and something different for those who study animal orientation.

Standardized and precise use of terms is, however, indispensable for analysis of the basic mechanisms controlling leukocyte locomotion under both experimental and clinical conditions. Such use of terms must allow for a clearcut distinction between:

(1) Description of forms of behaviour, such as random or directional locomotion on the one hand and the interpretation of these observations in terms of cell functions (intrinsic locomotor capacity, chemokinesis, chemotaxis, etc.) on the other.

(2) The intrinsic locomotor capacity of a cell on the one hand and reactions to regulatory environmental influences (chemokinesis and/or chemotaxis, etc.) on the other.

(3) Different types of reaction (chemokinesis, chemotaxis, etc.) to environmental influences.

The evaluation of terms currently used in biology to describe locomotion of cells or organisms shows that they permit such distinctions, provided the terms are used in a well defined and standardized way. The present proposals are mainly concerned with leukocytes because these cells show chemokinesis as well as chemotaxis and because the confusion of terms is particularly obvious in this field. The same criteria should however be applied to all cells or organisms. We believe that such a uniform scheme would encourage a more complete evaluation of cell behaviour and permit valid comparisons of the behaviour exhibited by different cells or organisms. In the following section, we present a proposal for such a standardized terminology with particular reference to responses to chemical stimuli and discuss the use of the different terms.

NOMENCLATURE

Definition of basic forms of locomotor behaviour

Random locomotion. A type of locomotion that is random in direction. The axis of the moving cell or organism is not oriented in relation to the stimulus.

NOTE. The term *random locomotion* (*12*, *13*) usually refers to motion in which the cell or organism shows a tendency to move along a path that can be represented by a line segment, but that is randomly oriented in relation to the environment. However, it can also refer to locomotion according to a random-walk model (*13*), in which—if the path of the cell is represented as a series of line segments meeting at angles—the spatial orientation and magnitude of each angle are determined solely by chance, and in which the mean square displacement of the cell is proportional to time.

Directional locomotion. Locomotion with preference for or avoidance of a particular direction. The axis of the migrating cells or organisms is oriented in relation to the stimulus.

Definition of some particular functions that influence cell locomotion

Intrinsic locomotor capacity. An intrinsic capacity of the cell to perform active locomotion.

NOTE. The expression of intrinsic locomotor capacity depends on other variables such as adhesion (*14*, *15*), detachment (*16*) of cells, and, conceivably, deformability (*17*, *18*).

Chemokinesis. A reaction by which the *speed* or frequency of locomotion of cells and/or the frequency and magnitude of *turning* (change of direction) of cells or organisms moving at random is determined by substances in the environment. Chemokinesis is said to be positive if displacement of cells moving at random is increased and negative if displacement is decreased.[a]

By analogy with chemotactic mediators (see below), chemokinetic mediators can be called cytokinesins or chemokinetic substances or factors.

Two forms of kinesis have been distinguished (*1*):

Orthokinesis, a reaction by which the speed or frequency of locomotion is determined by the intensity of the stimulus.

Klinokinesis, a reaction by which the frequency or the amount of turning per unit time is determined by the intensity of the stimulus.

Chemotaxis. A reaction by which the direction of locomotion of cells or organisms is determined by substances in their environment.

If the direction is towards the stimulating substance, chemotaxis is said to be positive, if away from the stimulating substance, the reaction is negative. If the *direction* of movement is not definitely towards or away from the substance in question, chemotaxis is indifferent or absent (*19*).

Positive chemotaxis can result in the cells being attracted towards the stimulating agent or in their being retained in high concentrations of the active substances by avoidance of low concentrations. Chemotaxis is increased when the directionality of locomotion is increased; if the directionality is decreased, chemotaxis is said to be decreased.

---

[a] This expresses the meaning of the term chemokinesis as first proposed by Rothert (*3*). The present formulation is based on McCutcheon's definition of chemotaxis (*19*) (see below).

Terms such as necrotaxis (*20*) have been proposed in order to characterize the source of the attractant. Chemotactic mediators have been termed cytotaxins (*21*) or more vaguely chemotactic substances (*22*) or factors (*23*).

APPLICATIONS OF TERMS

The terms that have been defined above should not be used unless the forms of behaviour they describe have been demonstrated experimentally. If the experimental data do not justify such a precise description, noncommital descriptive terms should be used. Where the only information is that cells have responded to an agent with increased movement, for instance increased penetration into the filter, noncommittal terms such as *stimulated movement* or *increased movement* should be employed (*24*).

Distinction between basic forms of locomotor behaviour and functions

None of the current methods of investigation provides for a direct measurement of functions such as intrinsic locomotor capacity, chemokinesis, or chemotaxis. These functions have to be determined by analysis of complex phenomena, such as random and/or directional locomotion.

Examples

- The fact that cells or organisms accumulate in response to a chemical gradient is not sufficient proof of directional migration or chemotaxis. The analysis of the behaviour of individual cells or organisms has shown that such a phenomenon can be due either to biased random locomotion in the form of klinokinesis (*25, 26, 27*) or to directional locomotion in the form of chemotaxis (*7, 19, 20*).
- Decreased cell displacement during random locomotion may reflect defects in its intrinsic locomotor capacity, due, for instance, to structural defects in the contractile system of the cell (*28*), or may indicate negative chemokinesis due to regulatory substances, such as neutrophil immobilizing factors (*29, 30*).
- Decreased cell displacement during directional locomotion may reflect defects in its intrinsic locomotor capacity or may indicate negative chemokinesis and/or decreased chemotaxis, e.g., due to "deactivation" with cytotaxins (*23*) or to cellular defects of chemotaxis (*4*).

Distinction between intrinsic locomotor capacity and reactions to environmental factors such as chemokinesis and chemotaxis

The distinction presents no problem if chemicals are evaluated for their activity on moving cells *in vitro*. It is also easy to distinguish changes in chemotaxis from altered intrinsic locomotor capacity by measuring random locomotion concomitantly. It is, however, more difficult to decide whether cells obtained from a patient show impaired locomotion because of intrinsic defects in the cell or due to immobilizing factors.

Examples

- If the behaviour of leukocytes from patients with the "lazy leukocyte" syndrome is analysed on the basis of the proposed terms it is found that they exhibit decreased random locomotion but no defect of chemotaxis (*6*).
- Cells may behave like "lazy leukocytes" because of intrinsic defects—for instance, in their contractile system (*28*)—or as a result of regulatory chemokinetic influences (*29, 30*). It is still uncertain which of these possibilities applies to the actual "lazy leukocyte" syndrome (*31*). In such a situation additional experiments are needed to evaluate cell adhesion, deformability, contractile structures, and metabolic processes in the "lazy leukocytes" or the presence of cytokinesins in the circulating blood of these patients.

Distinction between chemotaxis and chemokinesis

Experimental and clinical studies indicate that chemokinesis and chemotaxis can be regulated by different factors and mechanisms (*4, 19*). Exclusive assessment of cell accumulation in a chemical gradient does not make it possible to distinguish between chemotaxis and chemokinesis. However, if cell locomotion is oriented relative to the gradient axis, then chemotaxis is present. If the speed of locomotion or rate of change of direction is different in different parts of the gradient, then chemokinesis should also be suspected and this can be assessed separately at different concentrations of the factor in nongradient situations if the cells do not adapt to the stimulus or if adaptation is slow enough (*32, 33*). If they adapt to the stimulus within a very short time, chemokinesis can be demonstrated only in a concentration gradient.

Example

- Certain substances have been reported to be exclusively chemotactic in their effect (*19, 34*), while neutrophil-immobilizing factors (*29, 30*) can affect the rate of locomotion without exerting a chemotactic effect.

Annex

SCIENTISTS RESPONSIBLE FOR FORMULATING THE FOREGOING PROPOSAL

The original draft of the proposal was drawn up by H. U. Keller, P. C. Wilkinson, M. Abercrombie, E. L. Becker, J. G. Hirsch, M. E. Miller, W. S. Ramsey, and S. H. Zigmond, and was published in three journals:

Cell biology international reports, **1**: 391-397 (1977)
Clinical and experimental immunology, **27**: 377-380 (1977)
The journal of immunology, **121**: 2122-2124 (1978).

Following publication of the original proposal, comments and suggestions were received from a number of other scientists and these were taken into consideration in revising it to produce the version published above. This modified version has been agreed upon by the following scientists:

H. U. Keller, Bern, Switzerland; P. C. Wilkinson, Cambridge, England; M. Abercrombie, Cambridge, England; E. L. Becker, Farmington, USA; J. G. Hirsch, New York, USA; M. E. Miller, Torrance, USA; W. S. Ramsey, Corning, NY, USA; S. H. Zigmond, Philadelphia, USA; F. K. Austen, Boston, USA; J. Baum, Rochester, USA; J. F. Borel, Basle, Switzerland; A. S. G. Curtis, Glasgow, Scotland; G. A. Dunn, Cambridge, England; J. I. Gallin, Bethesda, USA; E. J. Goetzl, Boston, USA; A. K. Harris, Chapel Hill, USA; J. R. Humbert, Buffalo, USA; E. Sorkin, Davos-Platz, Switzerland; J. P. Trinkaus, New Haven, USA; J. M. Vasiliev, Moscow, USSR; L. Weiss, Buffalo, USA: J. H. Wissler, Bad Nauheim, Federal Republic of Germany.

REFERENCES

1. Fraenkel, G. S. & Gunn, D. L. *The orientation of animals. Kinesis, taxes and compass reactions.* London, Oxford University Press, 1940. Reprinted by Dover Publications, New York, 1961.
2. Pfeffer, W. Locomotorische Richtungsbewegung durch chemische Reize. *Untersuchungen aus dem botanischen Institut zu Tübingen,* **1**: 363-482 (1884).
3. Rothert, W. Beobachtungen und Betrachtungen über taktische Reizerscheinungen. *Flora,* **88**: 371-421 (1901).
4. Miller, M. E. *Pathology of chemotaxis and random mobility. Seminars in hematology,* **12**: 59-82 (1975).
5. Wilkinson, P. C. Cellular and molecular aspects of chemotaxis of macrophages and monocytes. *In*: Nelson, D. S., ed., *Immunobiology of the macrophage,* New York, Academic Press, 1976, pp. 349-365.
6. Keller, H. U. et al. Physiology of chemotaxis and random motility. *In*: Humbert, R. et al., ed., *Neutrophil physiology and pathology,* New York, Grune & Stratton, 1975, pp. 45-67.
7. Zigmond, S. H. Mechanisms of sensing chemical gradients by polymorphonuclear leucocytes. *Nature (London),* **249**: 450-452 (1974).
8. Keller, H. U. & Sorkin, E. Studies on chemotaxis. IV. The influence of serum factors on granulocyte locomotion. *Immunology,* **10**: 409-416 (1966).
9. Zigmond, S. H. & Hirsch, J. G. Leucocyte locomotion and chemotaxis. *Journal of experimental medicine,* **137**: 387-410 (1973).
10. Wilkinson, P. C. *Chemotaxis and inflammation.* Edinburgh & London, Churchill Livingstone, 1974.
11. Willmer, E. N. & Jacoby, F. Studies on the growth of tissues *in vitro*. IV. On the manner in which growth is stimulated by extracts of embryo tissues. *Journal of experimental biology,* **13**: 237-248 (1936).
12. Abercrombie, M. The locomotory behaviour of cells. *In* Willmer, E. N., ed., *Cells and tissues in culture,* London, Academic Press, 1965, vol. 1, pp. 177-202.
13. Gail, M. H. & Boone, CH. W. The locomotion of mouse fibroblasts in tissue culture. *Biophysical journal,* **10**: 980-993 (1970).
14. Wolpert, L. & Gingell, D. Cell surface membrane and amoeboid movement. *In*: *Symposium of the Society for Experimental Biology. XXII Aspects of Cell motility,* Cambridge, Cambridge University Press, 1968, pp. 169-198.
15. Trinkaus, J. P. The cellular basis of Fundulus epiboly. Adhesivity of blastula and gastrula cells in culture. *Developmental biology,* **7**: 513-532 (1963).
16. Weiss, L. & Glaves, D. Effects of migration inhibiting factor(s) on the in vitro detachment of macrophages. *Journal of immunology,* **115**: 1362-1365 (1975).
17. Miller, M. E. Developmental maturation of human neutrophil motility and its relationship to membrane deformability. *In*: Bellanti, J. A. & Dayton, D. H., ed., *The phagocytic cell in host resistance,* New York, Raven Press, 1975, pp. 295-307.
18. Tickle, C. & Trinkaus, J. P. Change in surface extensibility of fundulus deep cells during early development. *Journal of cell science,* **13**: 721-726 (1973).
19. McCutcheon, M. Chemotaxis in leukocytes. *Physiological reviews,* **26**: 319-336 (1946).
20. Bessis, M. & Burte, B. Positive and negative chemotaxis as observed after the destruction of a cell by U.V. or laser microbeams. *Texas reports on biology and medicine,* **23**: 204-212 (1965).

21. KELLER, H. U. & SORKIN, E. Studies on chemotaxis. V. On the chemotactic effect of bacteria. *International archives of allergy and applied immunology,* **31**: 505-517 (1967).
22. BOYDEN, S. The chemotactic effect of mixtures of antibody and antigen on polymorphonuclear leucocytes. *Journal of experimental medicine,* **115**: 454-466 (1962).
23. WARD, P. S. & BECKER, E. L. The deactivation of rabbit neutrophils by chemotactic factors and the nature of the activatable esterase. *Journal of experimental medicine,* **127**: 693-709 (1968).
24. SHOWELL, H. J. ET AL. The structure activity relations of synthetic peptides as chemotactic factors and inducers of lysosomal enzymes secretion for neutrophils. *Journal of experimental medicine,* **143**: 1154-1169 (1976).
25. BERG, H. C. & BROWN, D. A. Chemotaxis in *Escherichia coli* analysed by three-dimension tracking. *Nature (London),* **239**: 500-504 (1972).
26. TSANG, N. ET AL. Common mechanisms for repellents and attractants in bacterial chemotaxis. *Science,* **181**: 60-63 (1973).
27. GUNN, D. L. The meaning of the term "klinokinesis". *Animal behaviour,* **23**: 409-412 (1975).
28. BOXER, L. ET AL. Primary defect in neutrophil motility. *Clinical research,* **22**: 384 (1974).
29. GOETZEL, E. J. & AUSTEN, F. K. A neutrophil immobilizing factor derived from human leucocytes. I. Generation and partial characterization. *Journal of experimental medicine,* **136**: 1564-1580 (1972).
30. KELLER, H. U. ET AL. Studies on the regulation of the neutrophil chemotactic response using a rapid and reliable method for measuring random migration and chemotaxis of neutrophil granulocytes. *Agents and actions,* **6**: 326-339 (1976).
31. MILLER, M. E. ET AL. Lazy leucocyte syndrome. A new disorder of neutrophil function. *Lancet,* **1**: 665-669 (1971).
32. MACNAB, R. M. & KOSHLAND, D. E. The gradient-sensing mechanism in bacterial chemotaxis. *Proceedings of the National Academy of Sciences of the United States of America,* **69**: 2509-2512 (1972).
33. BROWN, D. A. & BERG, H. C. Temporal stimulation of chemotaxis in *Escherichia coli. Proceedings of the National Academy of Sciences of the United States of America,* **71**: 1388-1392 (1974).
34. RAMSEY, W. S. Analysis of individual leucocyte behaviour during chemotaxis. *Experimental cell research,* **70**: 129-139 (1972).

Allergen nomenclature*

This article presents a nomenclature system for allergens which has been officially recommended by the International Union of Immunological Societies (IUIS). The nomenclature is based on proposals of the IUIS Sub-Committee for Allergen Nomenclature and is applicable to highly purified, well-characterized allergens and to non-purified or partially purified allergenic extracts.

During the past several years, many antigens (allergens) which cause IgE-mediated atopic allergies in humans have been isolated from a wide variety of different sources. The number of nomenclature systems associated with these allergens has grown almost in proportion to the number of newly described components. In order to bring some order into the present, chaotic situation, the IUIS Sub-Committee for Allergen Nomenclature has proposed a new unified nomenclature system for (*a*) highly purified allergens and (*b*) individual components identified within complex allergenic mixtures by means of various immunochemical and physicochemical separation techniques. In the case of the highly purified allergens, the Sub-Committee also proposed guidelines for the criteria used to establish homogeneity, envisaging that the specialities of allergen chemistry in particular and of human immune response in general will benefit substantially through the exchange of reagents and data. Comparable practical benefits should also accrue in the area of allergen standardization.

Highly purified, well-characterized allergens (Table 1)

The source of the allergen will be clearly defined, including the accepted taxonomic name of the species and any further identification (e.g., strain designation, if appropriate). Where necessary, a physical description of the source material (e.g., fungal spores, 95% purity) and any processing of the source material will be included.

Highly purified allergens will be designated as follows: the first three letters of the genus (italicized); space; first letter of the species name (italicized); space; a Roman numeral. For example, *Lol p* I will refer to *Lolium perenne* allergen number one (perennial rye Group I (Rye I)). In the rare event that two species names have identical designations, they will be discriminated from one another by adding one or more letters (as necessary) to each species designation.

The allergens will usually be numbered in the order in which they were isolated, or by general agreement of the IUIS Nomenclature Sub-Committee. The following general exceptions apply:

(1) A major allergen will normally be assigned number one (e.g., *Amb a* I, short ragweed AgE; *Gad c* I, cod allergen M).

(2) Structurally homologous (but not necessarily cross-reactive) components from *different* species will be assigned the same numbers (e.g., *Der p* I, *Dermatophagoides pteronyssinus* P_1 and *Der f* I, *D. farinae* Ag11). This may require numbering certain allergens out of the sequence in which they were isolated or leaving gaps in the sequence of the numbers of allergens from certain species (e.g., as in the case of *Ambrosia trifida*, giant ragweed (Table 1)). It is also recognized that in exceptional cases, where homology is established after the initial nomenclature has been assigned, some revision of the

* This article is based on work that was supported by the U.S. National Institutes of Health (grants No. AI-19727, AI-17021 and AI-20565) and the Medical Research Council of Canada (grant No. MT-2010). All questions and comments and requests for reprints should be sent to Dr David G. Marsh, Chairman, IUIS Allergen Nomenclature Sub-Committee, Johns Hopkins University School of Medicine, The Good Samaritan Hospital, Division of Clinical Immunology, 5601 Loch Raven Blvd, Baltimore, MD 21239, USA.

Table 1. Examples of the nomenclature for some highly purified allergens

Source	New nomenclature	Old nomenclature
Grass pollens:		
Lolium perenne (perennial rye)	*Lol p* I	Group I (Rye I)
	Lol p II	Group II
	Lol p III	Group III
	Lol p IV	HMBA (GpIV?)
	Lol p X	Cytochrome c
Phleum pratense (timothy)	*Phl p* V	Ag25
	Phl p VI	Ag19
	Phl p VII	Ag30
	Phl p VIII	Ag3
Dactylis glomerata (orchard or cocksfoot)	*Dac g* I	Dg1
Poa pratensis (Kentucky blue; june)	*Poa p* X	Cytochrome c
Weed pollens:		
Ambrosia artemisiifolia (elatior) (short ragweed)	*Amb a* I	AgE
	Amb a II	AgK
	Amb a III	Ra5
	Amb a IV	Ra4(BPA-R)
	Amb a V*	Ra5
	Amb a VI	Ra6
Ambrosia trifida (giant ragweed)	*Amb t* V	Ra5G
Salsola pestifer (Russian thistle)	*Sal p* I	RT_1/RT_2
Tree pollens:		
Alnus incana (alder)	*Aln i* I	Al4
Betula verrucosa (silver birch)	*Bet v* I	Ag23(BV45?)
Corylus avellana (hazel)	*Cor a* I	Hla
Cryptomeria japonica (Japanese cedar)	*Cry j* I	SBP
House dust mites (*Dermatophagoides* spp.):		
D. pteronyssinus	*Der p* I	P_1(Ag42)
	Der p II	AgX
D. farinae	*Der f* I	Ag11(Ag6)
D. microceras	*Der m* I	Ag6
Non-biting midges (*Chironomus* spp.):		
C. thummi thummi	*Chi t* I	Haemoglobin[a]
Animal danders:		
Felis domesticus (cat)	*Fel d* I	Cat I(Ag4)
Equus caballus (horse)	*Equ c* I	Ag6
	Equ c II	Ag9
	Equ c III	Ag11
Bos domesticus (domestic cattle)	*Bos d* I	Ag1
	Bos d II	Ag3
	Bos d III	Ag6
Rattus norvegicus (rat)	*Rat n* I	prealbumin
	Rat n II	α_{2u}-globulin
Fungal spores:		
Alternaria alternata	*Alt a* I[b]	Alt-I(Ag1)
Cladosporium herbarum	*Cla h* I[b]	Ag32
	Cla h II[b]	Ag54
Hymenoptera venoms:		
Apis mellifera (honey bee)	*Api m* I	Phospholipase A_2
	Api m II	Hyaluronidase
	Api m III	Melittin
	Api m IV	Acid phosphatase
	Api m VI	Allergen C
Vespula germanica (yellow jacket)	*Ves g* I	Phospholipase A_1/B
	Ves g II	Hyaluronidase
	Ves g V	Ag5
Polistes annularis (wasp)	*Pol a* I	Phospholipase A_1/B
	Pol a II	Hyaluronidase
	Pol a V	Ag5
Ingestants:		
Gadus callarias (cod)	*Gad c* I	M (parvalbumin)
Gallus domesticus (chicken: egg white)	*Gal d* I	Ovomucoid
	Gal d II	Ovalbumin
	Gal d III	Conalbumin
Ascaris suum	*Asc s* I	Asc-1

[a] Eleven haemoglobins (erythrocruorins) of differing sequence, but highly cross-reactive, have been described in this species.
[b] ATCC No. to be added where appropriate (see text).

nomenclature may be necessary. (This may possibly be required in the case of the *Phleum pratense* (timothy) allergens).

(3) Homologous, immunologically closely related components within the same species (*isoallergens*) will be designated by capital letters (A,B,C, etc.) in the order of decreasing pI (e.g., *Amb a* VA, Ra5A (pI 9.6) and *Amb a* VB, Ra5B (pI 8.5)). If two closely related components have similar pI values (differing by less than 0.05 pI unit), they will be designated in the order of decreasing relative molecular mass, as determined by SDS-PAGE (sodium dodecyl sulfate

polyacrylamide gel electrophoresis) under reducing conditions,[a] or by more rigorous procedures such as sequence analysis (if not differentiated by SDS-PAGE).

The Sub-Committee recognizes that a few allergens, e.g., *Gal d* I (ovomucoid) and *Poa p* X (cytochrome c), already have been assigned biochemical names. In such cases, both the assigned allergen nomenclature and the biochemical name should first be specified and may be used interchangeably thereafter.

In the case of fungal allergens, where there is already evidence for strain differences within a species, the American Type Culture Collection (ATCC) number (or other appropriate numerical designation) will be included as a subscript after the allergen number, where it is necessary to designate such differences (e.g., *Alt a* I_{6663}, Alt-I isolated from *Alternaria alternata,* ATCC No. 6663, which is slightly different antigenically from *Alt a* I_{16086}). It is envisaged that a similar approach will be used in the future when strain or subspecies differences identified in other biological sources are described.

In regard to nomenclature, no attempt will be made to discriminate between components of different parts of the plant or animal source, nor between allergens that enter the body by different routes. The Sub-Committee appreciates that relatively clearly defined differences exist with respect to the route of exposure in certain cases (e.g., chicken eggs versus feathers), but in other cases (e.g., fish proteins) the route of sensitization may be by ingestion or inhalation, or by both of these routes.

Further abbreviated usage. Where reference is made to an allergen from a particular, clearly designated species (e.g., within a publication dealing with a single specified allergen source), the inclusion of the last italicized letter for the species will not be necessary (e.g., *Fel* I, cat allergen 1).

Purity requirements. In order to be designated according to the new system, the allergen must possess a high degree of purity according to several selected physicochemical and immunochemical criteria. At least four and preferably five different types of criteria are recommended, including (but not limited to) appropriate selection of separation techniques based on the following properties:

Molecular size: SDS-PAGE, gel filtration.

Molecular charge: Isoelectric focusing (IEF), electrophoresis (PAGE, agarose gel, starch gel, etc.), ion-exchange chromatography (especially high-performance liquid chromatography (HPLC) using an appropriate anionic or cationic exchanger).

Immunochemical: Crossed immunoelectrophoresis/crossed radioimmunoelectrophoresis (CIE/CRIE) or immunoelectrophoresis (IEP) using hyperimmune antisera from at least three outbred animals.

Hydrophobicity: Reverse-phase HPLC.

Chemical: NH_2-terminal amino acid determination, COOH-terminal amino acid determination, amino acid composition.

In each case, the experimental conditions should be clearly defined (see also footnote *a*).

It is recognized that closely related isoallergens are often not readily separable. In the case of isoallergenic mixtures, the pI and/or molecular size range will be specified.

Other requirements. The following physical and chemical parameters will be supplied where possible: relative molecular mass (under defined conditions; see also footnote *a*), amino acid composition and sequence, carbohydrate content and composition (as well as location and type of linkage if known), extinction coefficient (including conditions for measurement), nitrogen content, presence of prosthetic groups, enzymatic or other biological activity (if any), and X-ray crystallographic structure. Where appropriate international (and/or national) reference preparations are available, such as those produced through the IUIS-WHO allergen standardization programme, the investigator should provide a quantitative estimate of the content of the purified allergen in the reference; furthermore, in-house crude allergen preparations should also be standardized against the reference.

Each investigator should attempt to define the allergenic importance of the isolated allergen in a subpopulation of subjects who possess IgE antibody and/or react positively by skin test to a well-characterized, standardized extract or the crude allergenic mixture from which the purified allergen was derived. The allergic population studied should be clearly defined epidemiologically. In addition, the method

[a] Protein allergens having non-identical polypeptide chains which are held together by disulfide bonds and/or by non-covalent bonds, give multiple bands on SDS-PAGE under reducing conditions. In such cases, the relative molecular mass of a protein shall be the sum of its polypeptide chains required to form the monomeric protein unit as established by gel filtration or gel electrophoresis in the absence of denaturant.

of *in-vivo* and/or *in-vitro* testing used, and the criteria for positivity and quantitation of the degree of responsiveness, should be described.

The Sub-Committee further proposes that investigators should send their data and publications on highly purified allergens to the Chairman (Dr D. G. Marsh) in order that they may be made available to other investigators, and be periodically updated. It is envisaged that the availability of such a comprehensive record will be beneficial to researchers in many areas of human immune response and of atopic disease in particular.

Finally, and most importantly, the Sub-Committee recommends that each investigator reporting the purification of an allergen should, as a minimum requirement, be willing to supply a sufficient amount of a monospecific antibody (polyclonal or monoclonal) to selected qualified investigators in order to allow them to identify the allergen immunochemically.

Non-purified or partially purified allergenic extracts

CIE/CRIE and related technologies. Antigens (Ag) will be designated by Arabic numerals, starting with those showing greatest anodic mobility at pH 8.6 (e.g., *Cla h* Ag1, Ag2, etc.). Researchers should take care in defining the antisera used in CIE/CRIE and be willing to make the sera available to other laboratories in order to facilitate inter-laboratory comparisons.

IEF "immunoprinting" and related technologies where the pI is defined. Each IEF band (Bd) will be numbered according to its pI, rounded to the nearest 0.05 pI unit (e.g., *Dac g* Bd5.9).

SDS-PAGE and related technologies where the relative molecular mass is defined. Each band will be designated according to its relative molecular mass (e.g., *Der f* Bd17K), where the abbreviation "K" refers to "thousand".

Other points. The terminology used for CIE/CRIE will be kept distinct for that application. In the case of IEF and SDS-PAGE, where both the pI and relative molecular mass are known, the corresponding band may be designated using both types of data e.g., *Der f* Bd3.75/30K. The genus and/or species abbreviations may be omitted in a situation where there is no confusion concerning designation and where the species has been previously defined.

The Nomenclature Sub-Committee encourages collaborative efforts among investigators working with the same or a related species to exchange information and reagents in order to minimize confusing nomenclature differences between laboratories. The laboratory reference patterns obtained using the investigator's own reagents should be compared with those obtained using appropriate international or national reference preparations, where available. Highly purified allergens, covered under the standard nomenclature system, should also be identified in the reference patterns by the investigator, wherever possible. The Sub-Committee recommends that all defined, but not fully purified components (e.g., antigens recognized by CIE) should be investigated for allergenic activity (e.g., by CRIE) using at least 20-30 human sera from individuals who have high levels of IgE antibodies to the crude allergenic extract containing the defined component. Attempts should also be made to identify antigenically and allergenically cross-reactive components.

* * *

IUIS Sub-Committee for Allergen Nomenclature

David G. Marsh, Department of Medicine, Johns Hopkins University School of Medicine, The Good Samaritan Hospital, Baltimore, MD, USA (*Chairman*)

Lawrence Goodfriend, Faculty of Medicine, McGill University, Montreal, Quebec, Canada

Te Piao King, The Rockefeller University, New York, NY, USA

Henning Løwenstein, Protein Laboratory, University of Copenhagen, Copenhagen, Denmark

Thomas A. E. Platts-Mills, Division of Allergy and Clinical Immunology, Department of Internal Medicine, University of Virginia School of Medicine, Charlottesville, VA, USA

In addition to the Sub-Committee members, the following scientists have accepted the nomenclature system and will participate in a Committee-at-Large, which will periodically review the nomenclature:

Kjell Aas, Lars Aukrust, Brian A. Baldo, Xavier Baur, Lars Belin, Morten Borch, Martin D. Chapman, Jean-Pierre Dandeu, A. K. M. Ekramoddoullah, Said Elsayed, Erik Florvaag, Annette Ford, Donald R. Hoffman, Rabia Hussain, Henrik Ipsen, David G. Klapper, Tor Langeland, Samuel Lehrer, Peter Lind, Joan Longbottom, Terumasa Miyamoto, John L. Ohman, Jr, Gabriel Peltre, Marianne Roebber, Michael J. Schumacher, Alec Sehon, Gil Strejan, Keven J. Turner, Hogne Vik, Bent Weeke, Hiroshi Yasueda, and John W. Yunginger.

Allergen nomenclature*

IUIS/WHO Allergen Nomenclature Subcommittee[1]

The revised nomenclature for allergens is presented together with proposed nomenclatures for (a) *allergen genes, mRNAs and cDNAs, and* (b) *recombinant and synthetic peptides of allergenic interest.*

Introduction

Rapid advances have been made in the past few years on allergen characterization and sequence determination by chemical and molecular biological approaches. This is indicated by the list of allergens with known partial or complete amino acid sequences in Table 1. A number of other important allergens are known in addition to those in Table 1 but their sequences are as yet not known. A useful source for known allergens is the Allergen Database (ALBE) in which are compiled their known biochemical and immunological properties together with their sequence data if known (*1*).

To take into account these advances, a revision of the current allergen nomenclature system (*2*) is given below. As in the current nomenclature system, the proposed revisions are for allergens which induce IgE-mediated (atopic) allergy in humans. In addition to the expected thorough immunochemical characterization of any newly discovered allergen, investigators are urged to obtain partial, or preferably complete, sequence data before using the official nomenclature system. Also it is expected that investigators would screen a reasonable population size so as to establish the frequency of response in patients to the newly discovered allergens.

Investigators frequently refer to allergens as major or minor ones. The generally accepted meaning of this terminology is that an allergen is designated as either major or minor depending on whether greater or less than 50% of patients tested have the corresponding allergen-specific IgEs (cf. *3–5*).

The revised nomenclature for allergens is given below together with the proposed nomenclatures for (*a*) allergen genes, mRNAs and cDNAs and (*b*) recombinant and synthetic peptides of allergenic interest.

Revised nomenclature

(1) *Allergens*

Allergens are designated according to the accepted taxonomic name of their source as follows: the first three letters of the genus, space, the first letter of the species, space, and an Arabic number. The numbers are assigned to the allergens in the order of their identification, and the same number is generally used to designate homologous allergens of related species. As two examples, Lol p 1 refers to the first pollen allergen identified from *Lolium perenne*, rye grass, and Cyn d 1 refers to the homologous pollen allergen from *Cynodon dactylon*, Bermuda grass.

In some instances, the above system of the first 3 letters of a genus and the first letter of a species has to be modified to include an additional letter for designation of the exact genus or species. For example, 4 of the many vespids which can cause insect allergy are *Vespula vulgaris*, *Vespula vidua*, *Vespula consobrina* and *Vespa crabo*. The homologous major venom allergens, antigen 5s, from *Vespula vulgaris* and *Vespula vidua* are both designated as Ves v 5 in the existing nomenclature, and those from *Vespula consobrina* and *Vespa crabo* are designated as Ves c 5. To avoid these ambiguities, antigen 5s from *Vespula vulgaris* and *Vespula vidua* will be designated

* A résumé in French of this article appears on page 802. Requests for reprints should be addressed to the Chairman of the IUIS Nomenclature Committee, Professor Michel Kazatchkine, Unité d'Immunologie, Hôpital Broussais, 96 rue Didot, 75014 Paris, France.

[1] Members of this Nomenclature Subcommittee: Te Piao King (*Chairman*), Donald Hoffman, Henning Lowenstein, David G. Marsh, Thomas A.E. Platts-Mills and Wayne Thomas.

Reprint No. **5531**

Table 1: **Some allergens with known amino acid sequences**

Allergen source	Allergens; systematic and original names	MW (kDa)	Sequence data[a, b]	References[a]
A. Weed pollens				
Asterales				
Ambrosia artemisiifolia				
(short ragweed)	Amb a 1; antigen E	38	C	*8, 20*
	Amb a 2; antigen K	38	C	*8, 21*
	Amb a 3; Ra3	11	C	*22*
	Amb a 5; Ra5	5	C	*11, 23*
	Amb a 6; Ra6	10	C	*24, 25*
	Amb a 7; Ra7	12	P	*26*
	Amb a ?	11	C	*27*
Ambrosia trifida (giant ragweed)	Amb t 5; Ra5G	4.4	C	*9, 10, 28*
Artemisia vulgaris (mugwort)	Art v 2	35	P	*29*
B. Grass pollens				
Poales:				
Cynodon dactylon (Bermuda grass)	Cyn d 1	32	C	*30, 31*
Dactylis glomerata				
(orchard grass)	Dac g 1; AgDg1	32	P	*32*
	Dac g 2	11	C	*33*
	Dac g 5		P	*34*
Lolium perenne				
(rye grass)	Lol p 1; group I	27	C	*35, 36*
	Lol p 2; group II	11	C	*37*
	Lol p 3; group III	11	C	*38*
	Lol p 5	31	P	*34*
	Lol p 9; Lol p Ib	31/35	C	*39*
Phleum pratense				
(timothy)	Phl p 1	27	C	*40, 41*
	Phl p 5; Ag25	32	C	*42–45*
Poa pratensis				
(Kentucky blue grass)	Poa p 1; group I	33	P	*46*
	Poa p 5	31	P	*34*
	Poa p 9	32/34	C	*47*
Sorghum halepense (Johnson grass)	Sor h 1		C	*48*
C. Tree pollens				
Fagales:				
Alnus glutinosa (alder)	Aln g 1	17	C	*49*
Betula verrucosa				
(birch)	Bet v 1	17	C	*50*
	Bet v 2; profilin	15	C	*51*
Carpinus betulus (hornbeam)	Car b 1	17	C	*52*
Corylus avelana (hazel)	Cor a 1	17	C	*53*
Quercus alba (white oak)	Que a 1	17	P	*54*
Pinales:				
Cryptomeria japonica				
(sugi)	Cry j 1	41-45	C	*55, 56*
	Cry j 2		C	*57, 58*
Juniper sabinoides	Jun s 1		C	*59*

(Table 1: continued)

Juniper virginiana	Jun v 1		C	*58*
Oleales:				
Olea europea (olive)	Ole e 1		C	*59, 60*
D. Mites				
Dermatophagoides pteronyssinus (mite)	Der p 1; antigen P1	25	C	*61*
	Der p 2	14	C	*62*
	Der p 3; trypsin	28/30	P	*63*
	Der p 4; amylase	60	P	*64*
	Der p 5	14	C	*65*
	Der p 6; chymotrypsin	25	P	*66*
	Der p 7	22-28	C	*67*
Dermatophagoides microceras (mite)	Der m 1	25	P	*68*
Dermatophagoides farinae (mite)	Der f 1	25	C	*69*
	Der f 2	14	C	*70, 71*
	Der f 3	30	P	*72*
Lepidoglyphus destructor (storage mite)	Lep d ?	15	P	*73*
E. Animals				
Canis domesticus[c]	Can d 1		C	*74*
	Can d 2		C	*74*
Felis domesticus (cat saliva)	Fel d 1; cat-1	38	C	*15*
Mus musculus (mouse urine)	Mus m 1; MUP	19	C	*75, 76*
Rattus norvegius (rat urine)	Rat n 1	17	C	*77, 78*
F. Fungi				
Aspergillus fumigatus	Asp f 1	18	C	*79*
	Asp f ?	90	P	*80*
	Asp f ?	55	P	*81*
Candida albicans	Cand a ?	40	C	*82*
Alternaria alternata	Alt a 1	28	P	*83–85*
Trichophyton tonsurans	Tri t 1	30	P	*86*
G. Insects				
Apis mellifera (honey bee)	Api m 1; phospholipase A2	16	C	*87*
	Api m 2; hyaluronidase	44	C	88
	Api m 4; melittin	3	C	89
Bombus pennsylvanicus (bumble bee)	Bom p 1; phospholipase	16	P	*90*
	Bom p 4; protease		P	*90*
Blattaria germanica (cockroach)	Bla g 2	20	C	*91*
Chironomus thummi thummi (midges)	Chi t 1; hemoglobin	16	C	*92*
Dolichovespula maculata (white face hornet)	Dol m 1; phospholipase A1	35	C	*93*
	Dol m 2; hyaluronidase	44	C	*94*
	Dol m 5; antigen 5	23	C	*95, 96*
Dolichovespula arenaria (yellow hornet)	Dol a 5; antigen 5	23	C	*97*

(Table 1: continued)

Polistes annularis				
(wasp)	Pol a 1; phospholipase A1	5	P	*98*
	Pol a 2; hyaluronidase	44	P	*98*
	Pol a 5; antigen 5	23	C	*97*
Polistes exclamans				
(wasp)	Pol e 1; phospholipase A1	34	P	*100*
	Pol e 5; antigen 5	23	C	*97*
Polistes fuscatus				
(wasp)	Pol f 5; antigen 5	23	C	*99*
Polistes metricus				
(wasp)	Pol m 5; antigen 5	23	P	*99*
Vespula flavopilosa				
(yellowjacket)	Ves f 5; antigen 5	23	C	*99*
Vespula germanica				
(yellowjacket)	Ves g 5; antigen 5	23	C	*99*
Vespula maculifrons				
(yellowjacket)	Ves m 1; phospholipase A1	33.5	C	*101*
	Ves m 2; hyaluronidase	44	P	*102*
	Ves m 5; antigen 5	23	C	*97*
Vespula pennsylvanica				
(yellowjacket)	Ves p 5; antigen 5	23	C	*99*
Vespula squamosa				
(yellowjacket)	Ves s 5; antigen 5	23	C	*99*
Vespula vidua				
(wasp)	Ves vi 5	23	C	*99*
Vespula vulgaris				
(yellowjacket)	Ves v 1; phopholipase A1	35	C	*98*
	Ves v 2; hyaluronidase	44	P	*98*
	Ves v 5; antigen 5	23	C	*97*
Vespa crabo	Vesp c 1; phospholipase	34	P	*100*
	Vesp c 5.0101; antigen 5	23	C	*99*
	Vesp c 5.0102; antigen 5	23	C	*99*
Solenopsis invicta				
(fire ant)	Sol i 2	13	C	*103, 104*
	Sol i 3	24	C	*103*
	Sol i 4	13	C	*103*
H. Foods				
Gadus callarias				
(cod)	Gad c 1; allergen M	12	C	*105*
Gallus domesticus				
(chicken)	Gal d 1; ovomucoid	28	C	*106, 107*
	Gal d 2; ovalbumin	44	C	*106, 107*
	Gal d 3; conalbumin (Ag22)	78	C	*106, 107*
	Gal d 4; lysozyme	14	C	*106, 107*
Penaeus aztecus				
(brown shrimp)	Pen a 1	36	P	*108*
	Pen a 2; tropomyosin	34	P	*109*
Brassica juncea				
(oriental mustard)	Bra j 1; 25 albumin	14	C	*110*
Hordeum vulgare				
(barley)	Hor v 1; BMAI-1	15	C	*111*
Sinapis alba				
(yellow mustard)	Sin a 1; 25 albumin	14	C	*112*
I. Others				
Ascaris suum	Asc s 1	10	P	*113*
Hevea brasiliensis	Hev b 1; elongation factor	58	P	*114*

[a] References are those where partial (P) or complete (C) amino acid sequence data are available. Original references describing the initial characterization studies are not given because of limited space. We apologize to our colleagues whose allergen sequence data we may have overlooked for inclusion in this Table.
[b] Sequence data for group 5 and 9 allergens from several grass pollens indicate that they are highly homologous proteins. Comparison of complete sequence data of group 5 and 9 allergens from a single grass species will clarify whether these two groups are the same protein.
[c] *Canis domesticus* is also designated as *Canis familiaris.*

as Ves v 5 and Ves vi 5 respectively, and those from *Vespula consobrina* and *Vespa crabo* as Ves c 5 and Vesp c 5. In the examples given, the modified nomenclature is used for the allergens from *Vespula vidua* and *Vespa crabo*, as the allergens from *Vespula vulgaris* were characterized prior to those for *Vespula vidua* and *Vespa crabo*.

Another example is for allergens from the domestic dog (*Canis domesticus*) and the mold *Candida albicans*. To avoid ambiguity, the modified system is used to designate Can d and Cand a allergens from these two sources respectively.

In the current nomenclature system (*2*) the letters are italicized and the numerals are Roman numerals. In the revised system, only letters of normal type and Arabic numbers are used. The proposed changes conform to the accepted nomenclature used in bacterial genetics (*6*) and HLA system (*7*) in that italicized and normal characters are used to represent genotypes and phenotypes respectively.

(2) *Allergens and isoallergens*

An allergen from a single species may consist of several closely similar molecules. These similar molecules are designated as isoallergens when they share the following common biochemical properties: (*a*) similar molecular size; (*b*) identical biological function, if known, e.g. enzymatic action; and (*c*) >67% identity of amino acid sequences.

It is recognized that the recommended >67% sequence identity for 2 allergens to be assigned to the same group is only a guide. There are likely to be borderline cases. As an example, the ragweed allergens Amb a 1 and 2 share 65% amino acid sequence identity (*8*). These allergens were assigned to different groups because of their different immunochemical properties before their sequences were known.

Allergens from different species of the same or different genus which share the above-mentioned common biochemical properties are considered to belong to the same group and the sequence identity requirement can be <67% as is the case for allergens of the same species. For example, Amb a 5 and Amb t 5 from short and giant ragweed pollens have about 45% sequence identity (*9*), and also have similar tertiary structures (*10, 11*). Another example is the minor pollen allergens Amb a 10, Poa p 10 and Lol p 10 from ragweed (*12*), Kentucky bluegrass (*13*) and rye grass (*14*). Although their sequences are not known, they are assigned to the same allergen group as they clearly have the same biological function of cytochrome c.

(3) *Isoallergens and variants*

cDNA cloning of allergens often show nucleotide mutations which are either silent or which can lead to single or multiple amino acid substitutions. In the revised system, members of an allergen group which have >67% amino acid sequence identity are designated as isoallergens. Each isoallergen may have multiple forms of closely similar sequences, which are designated as variants.

Isoallergens and their variants belonging to the same allergen group are designated by suffixes of a period followed by four Arabic numerals. The first two numerals 01 to 99 refer to a particular isoallergen, and the two subsequent numerals 01 to 99 refer to a particular variant of a particular isoallergen designated by the preceding two numerals. In cases where there is only one known isoallergen but there are several variants, the system of a suffix of 4 numerals will still apply. These numerals will be chosen in the order of the identification of allergens and/or their cDNAs irrespective of the physicochemical properties of the allergens. In cases of silent mutations, there can be more than one suffix of 4 numerals designating the same allergen and in that case the suffix with the lowest number will be used to designate the allergen of interest.

The addition of suffixes of 4 numerals to designate isoallergens and their variants will permit their unambiguous designation. In many cases it is unnecessary to specify the isoallergen or variant and the corresponding suffixes may be deleted; for example, Bet v 1 represents any Bet v 1 allergen and Bet v 1.0101 represents variant number 1 of isoallergen Bet v 1. Two other examples of this nomenclature system are given below.

On cDNA cloning, Amb a I showed multiple polymorphic forms which differ from each other by 12-24% in their sequences (*8*). Four such forms of Amb a I are known and they are designated as Amb a 1.01, 1.02, 1.03 and 1.04. Each isoallergen of the Amb a I group is found to have 1 to 3 variants with >97% of sequence identity. These variants of the Amb a 1.01 group will be designated as Amb a 1.0101, 1.0102 and etc.

In contrast to Amb a I, only two forms of Amb a II were found on cDNA cloning. These forms differ in two polymorphic sites and they have >99% amino acid sequence identity. They are designated as Amb a 2.0101 and 2.0102.

Nomenclature for allergen genes, mRNAs and cDNAs

At present the genomic structures of allergens are known in at least two cases; cat allergen Fel d 1 and mouse urinary allergen Mus m 1. Knowledge of the genomic structure can provide an understanding of how the different polymorphic forms are generated by differential splicing and/or exon usage. By adopting the revised nomenclature for allergens, we can reserve the italicized characters to designate an allergen gene. Normal characters are used for designation of mRNAs and cDNAs.

For example, Fel d 1 is a protein consisting of two polypeptide chains (*15*) which are encoded by two separate genes (*16*). The two allergen genes for chains 1 and 2 of Fel d 1 will be represented by *Fel d 1A* and *Fel d 1B* respectively. Allelic forms of mRNAs and cDNAs of the *Fel d 1A* gene are designated as mRNA or cDNA Fel d 1A.0101 where the numerals are to correspond to those of the polymorphic allergens.

Nomenclature for recombinant and synthetic peptides of allergenic interest

There is interest in the possible use of fragments of allergens as reagents to modulate allergen-specific immune responses. Such fragments may be prepared by recombinant technology or by chemical synthesis. Therefore it is useful to establish a generally accepted nomenclature for such peptides of allergenic interest.

The nomenclature for recombinant and synthetic peptides of allergenic interest is to be based on the nomenclature for naturally occurring allergens since it is well accepted by the scientific and the clinical communities. An allergen which is prepared by recombinant (r) or chemical synthetic (s) means is to be differentiated from a natural (n) allergen by the addition of the prefix of r or s followed by a suffix of the amino acid residue positions which are given in parenthesis. For examples, a recombinant hornet venom allergen Dol m 5.0201 which contains the entire sequence of 204 residues will be designated as rDol m 5.0201, and a recombinant or synthetic peptide of residue 151-165 of Dol m 5.0201 will be designated as r or sDol m 5.0201 (151-165) respectively.

Natural allergens may contain post-translational modifications as many proteins do. These modifications include glycosylation, acylation, methylation, etc. Recombinant or synthetic allergen, designated by the prefix r or s, is taken to indicate that it does not contain the post-translational modification of the natural allergen. If the recombinant or synthetic allergen does contain the exact same modification as that of the natural allergen, it will be designated with a prefix of rn or sn. For example, the honey bee venom allergen phospholipase A2, Api m 1, is a glycoprotein with an oligosaccharide attached at the asparagine residue number 13 (*17, 18*). A synthetic peptide of residues 1-20 of Api m 1 without the oligosaccharide at residue 13 will be designated as sApi m 1 (1-20), and a synthetic peptide of residue 1-20 with the exact same oligosaccharide of the natural allergen will be designated as snApi m 1 (1-20).

For recombinant or synthetic fragments which are derivatives of sequences contained within the native allergen structure, an additional suffix enclosed in square brackets will be used to indicate that the peptide referred to is an analogue. Substitutions or modifications of amino acid residues are given with the standard one-letter code and superscript numbers indicate the residue positions at which modifications occur. The one-letter codes for L-amino acids are given in upper case letters and those for D-amino acids are in lower case letters. The modifications which can be substitution, insertion or deletion are specified in parenthesis within the brackets. Obviously when there are many changes, it will not be practical to follow this nomenclature but to give the fully modified sequences. Examples of these analogues of sDol m 5.0201 (151-165) are given below:

Unmodified: sDol m 5.0201 (151-165)

Substitution: sDol m 5.0201 (151-165) [K ^{153}]

— L-lysine residue at position 153 of sDol m 5.0201 (151-165) is substituted with D-lysine

Insertion: sDol m 5.0201 (151-165) [+K ^{153}]

— one residue of L-lysine is inserted between positions 153-154

Deletion: sDol m 5.0201 (151-165) [-K ^{153}]

— L-lysine residue at position 153 is deleted

N-terminal modification: sDol m 5.0201 (151-165) [N-Ac]

— *N*-terminal amino group is acetylated

C-terminal modification: sDol m 5.0201 (151-165) [C-NH_2]

— *C*-terminal carboxyl group is in the form of carboxamide

The nomenclature proposed above is very similar to that used for synthetic peptides representative of immunoglobulin sequences (*19*).

Acknowledgement

We thank Drs Martin Chapman, Irwin Griffith, Shayam Mohaptra, Rosalia Rodriguez and Alec Sehon for reviewing this article.

Résumé

Nomenclature des allergènes

La nomenclature des allergènes a été mise à jour en tenant compte des progrès rapides réalisés ces dernières années dans la caractérisation des allergènes et la détermination de leur séquence en acides aminés par des techniques biochimiques et de biologie moléculaire.

La nouvelle nomenclature est présentée dans un tableau concernant les allergènes, les isoallergènes et leurs variants (pollens, acariens, autres allergènes, animaux, mycophytes, insectes, aliments, divers). La nomenclature concerne également a) les gènes, les ARNm et les ADNc des allergènes et b) les peptides synthétiques et recombinants importants en allergologie.

References

1. **Marsh DG, Freidhoff LR.** *ALBE, An allergen database.* IUIS, Baltimore, MD, Edition 1.0.
2. **Marsh DG et al**. Allergen nomenclature. *Bulletin of the World Health Organization*, 1986, **64**: 767-770.
3. **King TP, PS Norman, Cornell JT.** Isolation and characterization of allergen from ragweed pollen. II. *Biochemistry*, 1964, **3**: 458-468.
4. **Lowenstein H.** Timothy pollen allergens. *Allergy*, 1980, **35**: 188-191.
5. **Aukrust L.** Purification of allergens in *Cladosporium herbarum. Allergy*, 1980, **35**: 206-207.
6. **Demerec M et al.** A proposal for a uniform nomenclature in bacterial genetics. *Genetics*, 1966, **54**: 61-75.
7. **Bodmer JG et al.** Nomenclature for factors of the HLA system, 1990. *Immunogenetics*, 1991, **33**: 301-309.
8. **Griffith IJ et al.** Sequence polymorphism of Amb a I and Amb a II, the major allergens in *Ambrosia artemisiifolia* (short ragweed). *Int. arch. allergy appl. immunol.*, 1991, **96**: 296-304.
9. **Roebber M et al.** Immunochemical and genetic studies of Amb t V (Ra5G), an Ra5 homologue from giant ragweed pollen. *J. immunol.*, 1985, **134**: 3062-3069.
10. **Metzler WJ et al.** Solution structures of ragweed allergen Amb t V. *Biochemistry*, 1992, **31**: 5117-5127.
11. **Metzler WJ et al.** Proton resonance assignments and three-dimensional solution structure of the ragweed allergen Amb a V by nuclear magnetic resonance spectroscopy. *Biochemistry*, 1992, **31**: 8697-8705.
12. **Goodfriend L et al.** Cytochromes C: new ragweed pollen allergens. *Federation proceedings*, 1979, **38**: 1415.
13. **Ekramoddoullah AKM, Kisil FT, Sehon AH.** Allergenic cross reactivity of cytochrome c from Kentucky bluegrass and perennial ryegrass pollens. *Mol. immunol.*, 1982, **19**: 1527-1534.
14. **Ansari AA, Killoran EA, Marsh DG.** An investigation of human response to perennial ryegrass (*Lolium perenne*) pollen cytochrome c (Lol p X). *J. allergy clin. immunol.*, 1987, **80**: 229-235.
15. **Morgenstern JP et al.** Amino acid sequence of Fel d I, the major allergen of the domestic cat: protein sequence analysis and cDNA cloning. *Proc. Natl Acad. Sci. USA*, 1991, **88**: 9690-9694.
16. **Griffith IJ et al.** Expression and genomic structure of the genes encoding FdI, the major allergen from the domestic cat. *Gene*, 1992, **113**: 263-268.
17. **Weber A, Marz L, Altmann F.** Characteristics of the asparagine-linked oligosaccharide from honeybee venom phospholipase A2. *Comp. biochem. physiol.*, 1986, **83B**: 321-324.
18. **Weber A et al.** Specific interaction of IgE antibodies with a carbohydrate epitope of honey bee venom phospholipase A2. *Allergy*, 1987, **42**: 464-470.
19. **Stanworth DR et al**. Nomenclature for synthetic peptides representative of immunoglobulin chain sequences. *Bulletin of the World Health Organization*, 1990, **68**: 109-111.
20. **Rafnar T et al.** Cloning of Amb a I (Antigen E), the major allergen family of short ragweed pollen. *J. biol. chem.*, 1991, **266**: 1229-1236.
21. **Rogers BL et al.** Complete sequence of the allergen Amb a II: recombinant expression and reactivity with T cells from ragweed allergic patients. *J. immunol.*, 1991, **147**: 2547-2552.
22. **Klapper DG, Goodfriend L, Capra JD.** Amino acid sequence of ragweed allergen Ra3. *Biochemistry*, 1980, **19**: 5729-5734.
23. **Ghosh B et al.** Cloning and expression of immunologically active recombinant Amb a V allergen of short ragweed (*Ambrosia artemisiifolia*) pollen. *J. immunol.*, 1993, **150**: 5391-5399.
24. **Roebber M et al.** Isolation and properties of a new short ragweed pollen allergen, Ra6. *J. immunol.*, 1983, **131**: 706-711.
25. **Lubahn B, Klapper DG.** Cloning and characterization of ragweed allergen Amb a VI (abst). *J. allergy clin. immunol.*, 1993, **91**: 338.
26. **Roebber M, Marsh DG.** Isolation and characterization of allergen Amb a VII from short ragweed pollen. *J. allergy clin. immunol.*, 1991, **87**: 324.
27. **Rogers BL et al.** Cloning, complete sequence, and recombinant expression of a novel allergen from short ragweed pollen (abst). *J. allergy clin. immunol.*, 1993, **91**: 339.
28. **Goodfriend L et al.** Ra5G, a homologue of Ra5 in giant ragweed pollen: isolation, HLA-DR-associated activity and amino acid sequence. *Mol. immunol.*, 1985, **22**: 899-906.
29. **Nilsen BM et al**. Structural analysis of the glycoprotein allergen Art v II from pollen of mugwort (*Artemesia vulgaris*). *J. biol. chem.*, 1991, **266**: 2660-2668.
30. **Matthiesen F, Schumacher M, Lowenstein H.** Characterization of the major allergen of *Cynodon dactylon* (Bermuda grass) pollen. *J. allergy clin. immunol.*, 1991, **88**: 763-774.
31. **Smith PM, Singh MB, Knox RB.** Characterization and cloning of the major allergen of Bermuda grass, Cyn d I. In: Kraft D, Sehon A. eds. *Molecular biology and immunology of allergens.* Boca Raton, CRC Press, 1993: 157-160.
32. **Mecheri S, Peltre G, David B.** Purification and characterization of a major allergen from *Dactylis glomerata* pollen: the Ag Dg 1. *Int. archs allergy appl. immunol.*, 1985, **78**: 283-289.
33. **Roberts AM et al**. Nucleotide sequence of cDNA

encoding the Group II allergen of Cocksfoot/-Orchard grass (*Dactylis glomerata*), Dac g II. *European j. allergy clin. immunol.*, 1993, In press.

34. **Klysner S et al.** Group V allergens in grass pollen IV. Similarities in amino acid compositions and amino terminal sequences of the group V allergens from *Lolium perenne, Poa pratensis and Dactylis glomerata. Clin. exp. allergy*, 1992, **22**: 491-497.

35. **Perez M et al.** cDNA cloning and immunological characterization of the rye grass allergen Lol p I. *J. biol. chem.*, 1990, **265**: 16210-16215.

36. **Griffith IJ et al.** Cloning and sequencing of Lol p I, the major allergenic protein of rye-grass pollen. *FEBS letters*, 1991, **279**: 210-215.

37. **Ansari AA, Shenbagamurthi P, Marsh DG.** Complete amino acid sequence of a *Lolium perenne* (perennial rye grass) pollen allergen, Lol p II. *J. biol. chem.*, 1989, **264**: 11181-11185.

38. **Ansari AA, Shenbagamurthi P, Marsh DG.** Complete primary structure of a *Lolium perenne* (perennial rye grass) pollen allergen, Lol p III: Comparison with known Lol p I and II sequences. *Biochemistry*, 1989, **28**: 8665-8670.

39. **Singh MB et al.** Isolation of cDNA encoding a newly identified major allergenic protein of rye-grass pollen: intracellular targeting to the amyloplost. *Proc. Natl Acad. Sci.*, 1991, **88**: 1384-1388.

40. **Matthiesen F et al.** NH2-terminal sequences of four immunoaffinity purified grass pollen allergens: Phl p I, Poa p I, Sec c I and Cyn d I (abst.). *Allergy* (Supp.), 1992, **47**: 31.

41. **Laffer S et al.** cDNA cloning of a major allergen of rye (*Secale cereale*) and timothy grass (*Phleum pratense*). *XVth Eur. Congress of Allergology and Clin. Immunol.*,1992, Paris.

42. **Matthiesen F, Lowenstein H.** Group V allergens in grass pollens. I. Purification and characterization of the group V allergen from *Phleum pratense* pollen, Phl p V. *Clin. exp. allergy*, 1991, **21**: 297-307.

43. **Vrtala S et al.** cDNA cloning of a major grass pollen allergen from timothy grass (*Phleum pratense*): identification as Phl p V, a protein with possible targeting to the amyloplast. *XVth Eur. Congress of Allergology and Clin. Immunol.*, 1992, Paris.

44. **Peterson A, Becker WM, Schlaak M.** Characterization of isoforms of the major allergen Phl p V by immunoblotting and microsequencing. *Int. arch. allergy immunol.*, 1992, **98**: 105-109.

45. **Bufe A et al.** Partial mRNA sequence of Phl p V. EMBL accession number X70942, 1993.

46. **Esch RE, Klapper DG.** Isolation and characterization of a major cross-reactive grass group I allergenic determinant. *Mol. immunol.*, 1989, **26**: 557-561.

47. **Olsen E et al.** Identification and characterization of the Poa p IX group of basic allergens of Kentucky bluegrass pollen. *J. immunol.*, 1991, **147**: 205-211.

48. **Avjioglu A, Singh M, Knox RB.** Sequence analysis of Sor h I, the group I allergen of Johnson grass pollen and it comparison to rye-grass Lol p I (abst). *J. allergy clin. immunol.*, 1993, **91**: 340.

49. **Breiteneder H et al.** Complementary DNA cloning and expression in *Escherichia coli* of Aln g I, the major allergen in pollen of alder (*Alnus glutinosa*). *J. allergy clin. immunol.*, 1992, **90**: 909-917.

50. **Breiteneder H et al.** The gene coding for the major birch pollen allergen Bet v I is highly homologous to a pea disease resistance response gene. *EMBO j.*, 1989, **8**: 1935-1938.

51. **Valenta R et al.** Profilins constitute a novel family of functional plant pan-allergens. *J. exp. med.*, 1992, **175**: 377-385.

52. **Larsen JN, Sturman P, Ipsen H.** PCR based cloning and sequencing of isogenes encoding the tree pollen major allergen Car b I from *Carpinus betulus*, hornbeam. *Mol. immunol.*, 1992, **29**: 703-711.

53. **Breiteneder H et al.** Four recombinant isoforms of Cor a I, the major allergen of hazel pollen. *Europ. j. biochem.*, 1993, **212**: 355-362.

54. **Ipsen H, Hansen BC.** The NH2-terminal amino acid sequence of the immunochemically partial identical major allergens of alder (*Alnus glutinosa*) Aln g I, birch (*Betula verrucosa*) Bet v I, hornbeam (*Carpinus betulus*) Car b I and oak (*Quercus alba*) Que a I pollens. *Molecular immunology*, 1991, **28**: 1279-1288.

55. **Taniai M et al.** N-terminal amino acid sequence of a major allergen of Japanese cedar pollen (Cry j I). *FEBS letters,* 1988, **239**: 329-332.

56. **Griffith IJ et al.** The cDNA cloning of Cry j I, the major allergen of *Cryptomeria japonica* (Japanese cedar) (abst). *J. allergy clin. immunol.*, 1993, **91**: 339.

57. **Sakaguchi M et al.** Identification of the second major allergen of Japanese cedar pollen. *Allergy*, 1990, **45**: 309-312.

58. **Griffith I.** Personal communication.

59. **Cardaba B et al.** Antibody response to olive pollen antigens: association between HLA class II genes and IgE response to Ole e I (abst). *J. allergy clin. immunol.*, 1993, **91**: 338.

60. **Villalba M et al.** Amino acid sequence of Ole e I, the major allergen from olive tree pollen (*Olea europaea*). *Europ. j. biochem.* In press.

61. **Chua KY, Stewart GA, Thomas WR.** Sequence analysis of cDNA encoding for a major house dust mite allergen, Der p I. *J. exp. med.*, 1988; **167**: 175-182.

62. **Chua KY et al.** Isolation of cDNA coding for the major mite allergen Der p II by IgE plaque immunoassay. *Int. arch. allergy appl. immunol.*, 1990, **91**: 118-123.

63. **Stewart GA et al.** The group III allergen from the house dust mite *Dermatophagoides pteronyssinus* is a trypsin-like enzyme. *Immunol.*, 1992, **75**: 29-35.

64. **Lake FR et al.** House dust mite-derived amylase: allergenicity and physicochemical characterisation. *J. allergy clin. immunol.* 1991, **87**: 1035-1042.

65. **Tovey ER et al.** Cloning and sequencing of a cDNA expressing a recombinant house dust mite protein that binds human IgE and corresponds to an important low molecular weight allergen. *J. exp. med.*, 1989, **170**: 1457-1462.

66. **Yasueda H et al.** Allergenic and proteolytic properties of fourth allergens from Dermatophagoides mites. In: *Dust mite allergens and asthma. Report*

of the 2nd International Workshop, Brussels, UCB Institute of Allergy, 1991: 63-64.
67. **Shen H-D et al**. Molecular cloning of a house dust mite allergen with common antibody binding specificities with multiple components in mite extracts. *Clin. exp. allergy*. In press.
68. **Lind P, Hansen OC, Horn N.** The binding of mouse hybridoma and human IgE antibodies to the major fecal allergen, Der p I of *D. pteronyssinus*. *J. immunol.*, 1988, **140**: 4256-4262.
69. **Dilworth RJ, Chua KY, Thomas WR**. Sequence analysis of cDNA coding for a major house dust allergen Der f I. *Clin. exp. allergy*, 1991, **21**: 25-32.
70. **Nishiyama C et al.** Determination of three disulfide bonds in a major house dust mite allergen, Der f II. *Int. arch. allergy immunol.*, 1993, **101**: 159-166.
71. **Trudinger M, Chua KY, Thomas WR.** cDNA encoding the major dust mite allergen Der f II. *Clin. exp. allergy*, 1991, **21**: 33-38.
72. **Heymann et al**. Antigenic and structural analysis of group II allergens (Der f II and Der p II) from house dust mites (*Dermatophagoides spp*). *J. allergy clin. immunol.*, 1989, **83**: 1055-1067.
73. **van Hage-Hamsten M et al**. N-terminal amino acid sequence of major allergen of the mite *Lepidoglyphus destructor* (abst). *J. allergy clin. immunol.*, 1993, **91**: 353.
74. **Konieczny A.** Personal communication.
75. **McDonald B et al**. A 29 amino acid peptide derived from rat alpha 2 euglobulin triggers murine allergen specific human T cells (abst). *J. allergy clin. immunol.*, 1988, **83**: 251.
76. **Clarke AJ et al**. Structure of mouse urinary protein genes: differential splicing configurations in the 3'-non-coding region. *EMBO j.*, 1984, **3**: 1045-1052.
77. **Longbottom JL.** *Characterization of allergens from the urines of experimental animals*. London, Macmillan, 1983: 525-529.
78. **Laperche Y et al.** Tissue-specific control of alpha 2u globulin gene expression: constitutive synthesis in submaxillary gland. *Cell*, 1983, **32**: 453-460.
79. **Arruda LK, Mann BJ, Chapman MD.** Selective expression of a major allergen and cytotoxin, Asp f I in *Aspergillus fumigatus*. *J. immunol.*, 1992, **149**: 3554-3559.
80. **Kumar A et al**. Isolation and characterization of a recombinant heat shock protein of *Aspergillus fumigatus*. *J. allergy clin. immunol.*, 1993, **91**: 1024-1030.
81. **Teshima R et al**. Isolation and characterization of a major allergenic component (gp55) of *Aspergillus fumigatus*. *J. allergy clin. immunol.*, 1993, **92**: 698-706.
82. **Shen HD et al**. The 40 kd allergen of *Candida albicans* is an alcohol dehydrogenase: molecular cloning and immunological analysis using monoclonal antibodies. *Clin. exp. allergy*, 1991, **21**: 675-681.
83. **Matthiesen F, Olsen M, Lowenstein H.** Purification and partial sequence of the major allergen of *Alternaria alternata*, Alt a 1. *J. allergy clin. immunol.*, 1992, **89**: 241.
84. **Curran IHA et al**. Purification and partial characterization of a low molecular weight antigen from *Alternaria alternata* (abst). *J. allergy clin. immunol.*, 1992, **89**: 283.
85. **Vijay HM et al**. A major antigen of *Alternaria alternata* with potential for safe and effective immunotherapy. *J. allergy clin. immunol.*, 1993, **91**: 826-828.
86. **Deuell B et al**. *Trichophyton tonsurans* allergen I. *J. immunol.*, 1991, **147**: 96-101.
87. **Kuchler K et al**. Analysis of the cDNA for phospholipase A2 from honey bee venom glands: the deduced amino acid sequence reveals homology to the corresponding vertebrate enzymes. *Eur. j. biochem.*, 1989, **184**: 249-254.
88. **Gmachl M, Kreil G**. Bee venom hyaluronidase is homologous to a membrane protein of mammalian sperm. *Proc. Natl Acad. Sci. USA*, 1993, **90**: 3569-3573.
89. **Habermann E.** Bee and wasp venoms. *Science*, 1972, **177**: 314-322.
90. **Jacobson RS, Hoffman DR.** Characterization of bumblebee venom allergens (abst). *J. allergy clin. immunol.*, 1993, **91**: 187.
91. **Arruda LK, Vailes LD, Chapman MD.** Molecular cloning of cockroach (*B. germanica*) allergens (abst). *J. allergy clin. immunol.*, 1993, **91**: 188.
92. **Mazur G, Baur X, Liebers V.** Hypersensitivity to hemoglobins of the Diptera family Chironomidae: structural and functional studies of their immunogenic/allergenic sites. *Monog. allergy*, 1990, **28**: 121-137.
93. **Soldatova L, Kochoumian L, King TP.** Sequence similarity of a hornet (*D. maculata*) venom allergen phospholipase A1 with mammalian lipases. *FEBS letters*, 1993, **320**: 145-149.
94. **Lu G, Kochoumian L, King TP.** White face hornet venom allergen, hyaluronidase: cloning and its sequence similarity with other proteins (abst.). 1994. *J. allergy clin. immunol.*, **93**: 224.
95. **Fang KSF et al**. cDNA cloning and primary structure of a white-faced hornet venom allergen, antigen 5. *Proc. Natl Acad. Sci., USA*, 1988, **85**: 895-899.
96. **King TP et al**. Structural studies of a hornet venom allergen antigen 5, Dol m V and its sequence similarity with other proteins. *Protein sequences and data analysis*, 1990, **3**: 263-266.
97. **Lu G et al**. Sequence analysis and antigen cross reactivity of a venom allergen antigen 5 from hornets, wasps and yellowjackets. *J. immunol.*, 1993, **150**: 2823-2830.
98. **King TP**. 1992. Unpublished data.
99. **Hoffman DR.** Allergens in hymenoptera venom XXV: The amino acid sequences of antigen 5 molecules and the structural basis of antigenic cross-reactivity. *J. allergy clin. immunol.*, 1993, **92**: 707-716.
100. **Hoffman DR.** 1992. Unpublished data.
101. **Hoffman DR.** The complete amino acid sequence of a yellowjacket venom phospholipase (abst). *J. allergy clin. immunol.*, 1993, **91**:187.
102. **Jacobson RS, Hoffman DR, Kemeny DM.** The cross-reactivity between bee and vespid hyaluronidases has a structural basis (abst). *J. allergy clin. immunol.*, 1992, **89**: 292.
103. **Hoffman DR.** Allergens in Hymenoptera venom

XXIV: The amino acid sequences of imported fire ant venom allergens Sol i II, Sol i III, and Sol i IV. *J. allergy clin. immunol.*, 1993, **91**: 71-78.

104. **Schmidt M et al**. Nucleotide sequence of cDNA encoding the fire ant venom protein Sol i II. *FEBS letters*, 1993, **319**: 138-140.

105. **Elsayed S et al**. The allergenic structure of allergen M from cod. Tryptic peptides of fragment TM1. *Int. arch. allergy appl. immunol.*, 1976, **52**: 59-63.

106. **Hoffman DR.** Immunochemical identification of the allergens in egg white. *J. allergy clin. immunol.*, 1983, **71**: 481-486.

107. **Langeland T.** A clinical and immunological study of allergy to hen's egg white. IV. specific IgE antibodies to individual allergens in hen's egg white related to clinical and immunolgical parameters in egg-allergic patients. *Allergy*, 1983, **38**: 493-500.

108. **Daul DB et al.** Common crustacea allergens: identification of B cell epitopes with the shrimp specific monoclonal antibodies. In: Kraft D, Sehon A, eds. *Molecular biology and immunology of allergens.* Boca Raton, CRC Press, 1993: 291-293.

109. **Rao PVS et al**. Tropomyosin is the major shrimp allergen (abst). *J. allergy clin. immunol.*, 1993, **91**: 341.

110. **Monsalve RI et al**. Characterization of a new mustard allergen, Bra j IE. Detection of an allergenic epitope. *Biochem. j.,* 1993, **293**: 625-632.

111. **Mena MR et al**. A major barley allergen associated with baker's asthma disease is a glycosylated monomeric inhibitor of insect a-amylase: cDNA cloning and chromosomal location of the gene. *Plant molec. biol.*, 1992, **20**: 451-458.

112. **Menendez-Arias L et al**. Primary structure of the major allergen of yellow mustard (*Sinapis alba* L.) seed, *Sin a I. Eur. j. biochem.*, 1988, **177**: 159-166.

113. **Christie JF et al**. N-terminal amino acid sequence identity between a major allergen of *Ascaris lumbricoides* and *Ascaris suum* and MHC-restricted IgE responses to it. *Immunology*, 1990, **69**: 596-602.

114. **Czuppon AB et al**. The rubber elongation factor of rubber trees (*Hevea brasiliensis*) is the major allergen in latex. *J. allergy clin. immunol.*, 1993, **92**: 690-697.

Nomenclature of amyloid and amyloidosis*

WHO-IUIS Nomenclature Sub-Committee[1]

This classification of amyloid and amyloidosis is based on the amyloid fibril proteins, followed by a designation of the fibril protein precursor. Additional information includes the protein type or variant (where applicable) and the clinical diagnosis.

Main principles

When possible, the basis for nomenclature and classification of a case of amyloidosis under examination should be the fibril protein making up the amyloid deposits. In many instances, the amyloid fibril proteins are identical with or derived from intact fragments of proteins present in the serum. Such fibril protein precursors should be listed as a second set of data. In cases where the given amyloid protein exists in the form of different types or variants, this should be given as additional information when necessary. A fourth type of information is a description of the disease process affecting the patient (Table 1).

Amyloid proteins

Amyloid and amyloidosis should therefore be classified by the fibril protein. Only proteins which have been characterized by their amino acid sequence and are known to be integrated in the amyloid fibrils should be listed (Table 1). Extrafibrillar proteins, like protein AP (the amyloid P-component), although regularly present in amyloid deposits, are thus excluded. The protein designations and abbreviations are chosen using those accepted in the relevant fields of medicine and the basic sciences. They should also be recognized and understood by clinicians, students, etc.

The capital letter A (for amyloid) should be used as the first letter of all designations for amyloid proteins, followed by the protein designation in abbreviated form without any space after this first letter A. When a given term is abbreviated to one single letter, this should be a capital Roman letter or Greek lower-case letter, e.g., AA, Aβ. When a term is abbreviated into an acronym, e.g., transthyretin to TTR, all letters are capitalized. When the spelling of the term is maintained but the word is abbreviated, only the first letter is capitalized (e.g., cystatin to Cys).

Regarding numbers, both arabic and roman numerals are used in accord with the abbreviations/designations widely and traditionally accepted in the scientific world. Subscripts or superscripts are not used in order to simplify typing and use of word processing.

Aβ and β protein precursor (βPP) are designations for the fibril protein and its precursor in Alzheimer's disease, etc. (Table 1). The recently discovered amyloid fibril protein in the immunoglobulin heavy chain has been given the designation AH (*3*).

Protein precursor

The term protein precursor (Table 1) refers to the protein from which the actual amyloid fibril protein

---

* This article was drafted by the following group of experts: G. Husby (Norway (*Chairman*), S. Araki (Japan), E.P. Benditt (USA), M.D. Benson (USA), A.S. Cohen (USA), B. Frangione (USA), G.G. Glenner (USA), J.B. Natvig (Norway), and P. Westermark (Sweden). The document has been approved by the Nomenclature Committee of IUIS. A French translation appears on pages 109–112.

[1] Requests for reprints and all correspondence should be addressed to the Chairman of the IUIS Nomenclature Committee, Professor Michel D. Kazatchkine, Unité d'Immunopathologie, Hôpital Broussais, 96 rue Didot, 75014 Paris, France.

Reprint No. **5361**

Table 1: **Nomenclature and classification of amyloid and amyloidosis**

Amyloid protein [a, b]	Protein precursor	Protein type or variant	Clinical diagnosis	Reference
AA	apoSAA		Reactive (secondary) amyloidosis	*4–7*
			Familial Mediterranean fever	*8*
			Familial amyloid nephropathy with urticaria and deafness (Muckle-Wells' syndrome)	*9*
AL	κ, λ e.g., κIII	Aκ, Aλ, e.g., AκIII	Idiopathic (primary) amyloidosis, associated with myeloma or macroglobulinaemia	*10, 11*
AH	IgG 1 (γ1)	Aγ1		*3*
ATTR	Transthyretin	e.g., Met 30 [c]	Familial amyloid polyneuropathy, Portuguese	*12–15*
		e.g., Met III	Familial amyloid cardiomyopathy, Danish	*16*
		TTR or Ile 122	Systemic senile amyloidosis	*17, 18*
AApoAI	apoAI	Arg 26	Familial amyloid polyneuropathy, Iowa	*19*
AGel	Gelsolin	Asn 187 [d] (15)	Familial amyloidosis, Finnish	*20, 21*
ACys	Cystatin C	Gln 68	Hereditary cerebral hemorrhage with amyloidosis, Icelandic	*22*
Aβ	β protein precursor e.g., βPP 695 [e]	Gln 618 (22)	Alzheimer's disease	*23, 24*
			Down syndrome	
			Hereditary cerebral haemorrhage with amyloidosis, Dutch	*25*
Aβ2M	β2-microglobulin		Associated with chronic dialysis	*26, 27*
AScr	Scrapie protein precursor 33–35 [f] cellular form	Scrapie protein 27–30	Creutzfeldt-Jakob disease, etc.	*28*
		e.g., Leu 102	Gerstmann-Straüssler-Scheinker syndrome	*29*
ACal	(Pro)calcitonin	(Pro)calcitonin	In medullary carcinomas of the thyroid	*30*
AANF	Atrial natriuretic factor		Isolated atrial amyloid	*31*
AIAPP	Islet amyloid polypeptide		In islets of Langerhans Diabetes type II, insulinoma	*32*
AIns [g]	Insulin		Islet amyloid in the degu (a rodent)	*33*
AApoAII [g]	apoAII (murine)	Gln5	Amyloidosis in senescence, accelerated mice	*34*

[a] Non-fibrillar proteins, e.g., protein AP (amyloid P-component) excluded.
[b] Abbreviations: AA, amyloid A protein; SAA, serum amyloid A protein; apo, apolipoprotein; L, immunoglobulin light chain; H, immunoglobulin heavy chain.
[c] ATTR Met 30 when used in text.
[d] Amino acid position in the mature precursor protein. The position in the amyloid fibril protein is given in parentheses.
[e] Number of amino acid residues.
[f] Molecular mass (kilodaltons).
[g] Not found in humans.

(normal or variant) is thought to be derived. With the exception of β protein precursor these amyloid-related proteins can be demonstrated in serum, and in many cases the amyloid protein is a fragment, i.e., an incomplete degradation product of its precursor.

Protein type or variant

These represent a variety of classes and variable subgroups of immunoglobulins, molecular variant related to inherited amyloidoses, and a prohormone (i.e., procalcitonin). Class designation of immunoglobulin chains are given in Greek lower-case letter, gamma-chain subclass in Arabic numerals, and variable subgroups in Roman numerals.

The (single) amino acid substitutions in transthyretin and other proteins that account for the inherited amyloid protein variants are indicated by the amino acid that substitutes for the normal one using the 3-letter code, following one open space after the protein designation. This is followed by a single open space, again followed by the position in the protein (i.e., residue number from the *N*-terminal) in the respective intact, normal protein where the substitution occurs, e.g., ATTR Met 30. The number of the variant amino acid relates to that in the mature (native) precursor protein, whereas the position in the corresponding amyloid protein, which is a fragment of the precursor, is given in parentheses.

The Table shows only one example of protein type or variant for each amyloid protein. The only exception is TTR, where 3 different variants are related to different clinical forms of inherited amyloid disease. In the cases of multiple protein types or variants (i.e., immunoglobulins, TTR, Scrapie protein) "sub-tables" should be designed to include all those known at the present time.

Clinical descriptions

The clinical descriptions used in the Table are those traditionally used in clinical practice up to now. No attempt has been made to revise them except that the Roman numbers used to classify various familial amyloid polyneuropathies have been omitted, and replaced by the geographic origin of the actual families.

Because the fibril protein in many forms of amyloidosis is not known, and because only few examples of amyloid protein variants or subtypes are given in the Table, some clinical forms of amyloidosis are not listed.

Finally, it should be noted that the distinction between systemic and localized (organ or tissue-limited) amyloidoses has been avoided. This is because some amyloid deposits, which appear to be localized, may represent a predilection site of systemic amyloidosis.

References

1. **Cohen, A.S. et al.** In: Wegelius, O. & Pasternack, A., ed. *Amyloidosis*. London, Academic Press, 1975, p. IX.
2. **Benditt, E.P. et al.** Guidelines for nomenclature. In: Glenner, G.G. et al., ed. *Amyloid and amyloidosis*. Amsterdam, Excerpta Medica, 1980, pp. XI-XII.
3. **Eulitz, M. et al.** In: Natvig, J.B. et al., ed. *Amyloid and amyloidosis*. Dordrecht, Kluwer Academic Publishers, 1990.
4. **Benditt, E.P. et al.** The major proteins of human and monkey amyloid substance: common properties including unusual *N*-terminal amino acid sequences. *FEBS letters*, **19**: 169–173 (1971).
5. **Levin, M. et al.** Immunologic studies of the major non-immunoglobulin protein of amyloid. I. Identification and partial characterization of a related serum component. *J. exp. med.*, **138**: 373–380 (1973).
6. **Husby, G. et al.** Unique amyloid subunit common to different types of amyloid fibril. *Nature*, **244**: 362–364 (1973).
7. **Parmelee, D.C. et al.** Amino acid sequence of amyloid-related apoprotein (apo SAA1) from human high-density lipoprotein. *Biochemistry*, **21**: 3298–3303 (1972).
8. **Levin, M. et al.** The amino acid sequence of a major non-immunoglobulin component of some amyloid fibrils. *J. clin. invest.*, **51**: 2773–2776 (1972).
9. **Linke, R.P. et al.** Identification of amyloid A protein in a sporadic Muckle-Wells syndrome. *N*-terminal amino acid sequence after isolation from formalin-fixed tissue. *Lab. invest.*, **48**: 698–704 (1983).
10. **Glenner, G.G. et al.** An amyloid protein: the amino-terminal variable fragment of an immunoglobulin light chain. *Biochem. biophys. res. comm.*, **41**: 1287–1289 (1970).
11. **Glenner, G.G. et al.** Amyloid fibril proteins: proof of homology with immunoglobulin light chains by sequence analysis. *Science*, **172**: 1150–1151 (1971).
12. **Costa, P.P. et al.** Amyloid fibril protein related to pre-albumin familial amyloidotic polyneuropathy. *Proc. Natl Acad. Sci. USA*, **75**: 4499–4503 (1978).
13. **Tawara, S. et al.** Identification of amyloid pre-albumin variant in familial amyloidotic polyneuropathy (Japanese type). *Biochem. biophys. res. comm.*, **116**: 880–888 (1983).
14. **Francis, E. et al.** Polymorphism of human plasma thyroxin binding pre-albumin. *Biochem. biophys. res. comm.*, **114**: 657–662 (1983).
15. **Saraiva, M.J.M. et al.** Amyloid fibril protein in familial amyloidotic polyneuropathy (Porguguese type): definition of molecular abnormality in transthyretin (prealbumin). *J. clin. invest.*, **74**: 104–119 (1984).
16. **Nordlie, M. et al.** A new pre-albumin variant in familial amyloid cardiomyopathy of Danish origin. *Scand. j. immunol.*, **27**: 119–122 (1988).
17. **Gorevic, P.D., et al.** Systemic senile amyloidosis. Identification of a new pre-albumin (transthyretin)

variant in cardiac tissue: immunologic and biochemical similarity to one form of familial amyloidotic polyneuropathy. *J. clin. invest.*, **83**: 836–843 (1989).

18. **Westermark, P. et al.** Fibril in senile systemic amyloidosis is derived from normal transthyretin. *Proc. Natl Acad. Sci. USA*, **87**: 2843–2845 (1990).
19. **Nichols, W.C. et al.** Variant apolipoprotein A1 as a major constituent of a human hereditary amyloid. *Biochem. biophys. res. comm.*, **156**: 762–768 (1988).
20. **Maury, C.P.J. et al.** Finnish hereditary amyloidosis: amino acid sequence homology between the amyloid fibril protein and human plasma elsoline. *FEBS letters*, **260**: 85–87 (1990).
21. **Haltia, M. et al.** Amyloid protein in familial amyloidosis (Finnish type) is homologous to gelsolin, an actin-binding protein. *Biochem. biophys. res. comm.*, **167**: 927–932 (1990).
22. **Ghiso, J. et al.** Amyloid fibrils in hereditary cerebral hemorrhage with amyloidosis of Icelandic type is a variant of gamma-trace basic protein (cystatin C). *Proc. Natl Acad. Sci. USA*, **83**: 2974–2978 (1986).
23. **Glenner, G.G. & Wong, C.W.** Alzheimer's disease: initial report of the purification and characterization of a novel cerebrovascular amyloid protein. *Biochem. biophys. res. comm.*, **120**: 885–890 (1984).
24. **Glenner, G.G.** Alzheimer's disease: its proteins and genes. *Cell*, **82**: 307–308 (1988).
25. **Levy, E. et al.** Mutation of the Alzheimer's disease amyloid gene in hereditary cerebral hemorrhage. *Science*, **248**: 1124–1126 (1990).
26. **Gejyo, F. et al.** A new form of amyloid protein associated with chronic hemodialysis identified as beta-2 microglobulin. *Biochem. biophys. res. comm.*, **129**: 701–706 (1985).
27. **Gorevic, P.D. et al.** Beta-2 microglobulin is an amyloidogenic protein in man. *J. clin. invest.*, **76**: 2425–2429 (1985).
28. **Prusiner, S.B. et al.** Purification and structural studies of a major Scrapie prion protein. *Cell.*, **38**: 127–134 (1984).
29. **Hsiao, K. et al.** Linkage of a prion protein missense variant to Gerstmann-Straussler syndrome. *Nature*, **338**: 342–345 (1989).
30. **Sletten, K. et al.** Characterization of amyloid fibril proteins from medullary carcinoma of the thyroid. *J. exp. med.*, **143**: 993–998 (1976).
31. **Johansson, B. et al.** Atrial natriuretic peptide deposited as atrial amyloid fibrils. *Biochem. biophys. res. comm.*, **148**: 1087–1092 (1987).
32. **Westermark, P. et al.** A novel peptide in the calcitonin gene-related peptide family as an amyloid fibril protein in the endocrin pancreas. *Biochem. biophys. res. comm.*, **140**: 827–831 (1986).
33. **Hellman, U. et al.** Amino acid sequence from degu islet amyloid derived insulin shows unique sequence characteristics. *Biochem. biophys. res. comm.*, **169**: 571–577 (1990).
34. **Higuchi, K. et al.** The single proline-glutamine substitution at position 5 enhances the potency of amyloid fibril formation of murine ap. A-II. *FEBS letters*, **207**: 23–27 (1986).

The Immunologist

Editor in Chief
Jacob B. Natvig
Institute of Immunology and Rheumatology
Fr. Qvamsgt. 1
N-0172 Oslo
Norway
Tel.: +47 22 869690
Fax: +47 22 200636
E-mail: j.b.natvig@rh.uio.no

Associate Editor in Chief
Jacinta Kelly
Dept. of Biological Sciences
Dublin Institute of Technology
Kevin Street
Dublin 8, Ireland
Tel.: +353 1 402-4753
Fax: +353 1 402-4983
E-mail: jacinta.kelly@dit.ie

Publisher
Hogrefe & Huber Publishers
Seattle · Toronto · Bern · Göttingen

SUBSCRIPTION INFORMATION

The Immunologist is published 6 times per year. Subscriptions are available on an annual volume basis. To receive a sample copy, or to order a subscription, please contact the Publisher at one of the addresses given below. Payment may be made by check or international money order (in US $, Deutsche Mark, or pounds sterling), or by credit card (please supply details).

Subscription rates (1999)			
Libraries/Institutions	US $78.00	DM 139.00	£50.00
Individuals	US $68.00	DM 119.00	£43.00
Members	US $44.00	DM 74.00	£29.00
Postage & handling	US $ 6.00	DM 10.00	£ 3.50

To order, or to request a sample copy, contact one of the addresses given below.

CONTACT ADDRESSES

USA:
Hogrefe & Huber Publishers
PO Box 2487
Kirkland, WA 98083
Tel.: (425) 820-1500
Fax: (425) 823-8324
E-mail: hh@hhpub.com

Rest of the World:
Hogrefe & Huber Publishers
Rohnsweg 25, D-37085 Göttingen
Germany
Tel.: +49 551 496090
Fax: +49 551 4960988
E-mail: hhpub@hogrefe.de

Contents

The Immunologist Volume 6, Issues 1–4, 1998

(Issues 5 and 6 in press)

EDITORIALS

RESEARCH TRENDS

Clinical Trends

Horizons

Contents

The Immunologist
Volume 5, Issues 1–6, 1997